Is the vegetarian life for you? When you're well-informed about health, nutrition, and ethical and environmental issues, you can choose wisely—and incorporate your dietary choice into a healthy, happy lifestyle. *The Vegetarian Life* not only includes information on everything from the historical roots of vegetarianism to the nutritional guidelines you need to be aware of, but also offers a wide variety of easy-to-make meatless recipes for . . .

- egg drop soup
- cold pasta salad
- vegan vegetable lasagna
- potato pie
- cheese tortellini with red peppers and rosemary
  and more

THE
VEGETARIAN
LIFE

THE
VEGETARIAN
LIFE

How to Be a Veggie in a
Meat-Eating World

ELIZABETH
FERBER '88

B
BERKLEY BOOKS, NEW YORK

The names of the people who have told their stories about vegetarianism have been changed to protect their privacy.

THE VEGETARIAN LIFE

A Berkley Book / published by arrangement with the author

PRINTING HISTORY
Berkley edition / February 1998

All rights reserved.
Copyright © 1998 by Elizabeth Ferber.
Book design by Erin Lush.
This book may not be reproduced in whole
or in part, by mimeograph or any other means,
without permission. For information address:
The Berkley Publishing Group, a member of Penguin Putnam Inc.,
200 Madison Avenue, New York, New York 10016.

The Putnam Berkley World Wide Web site address is
http://www.berkley.com

ISBN: 0-425-15976-0

BERKLEY®
Berkley Books are published by The Berkley Publishing Group,
a member of Penguin Putnam Inc.,
200 Madison Avenue, New York, New York 10016.
BERKLEY and the "B" design are trademarks belonging to
Berkley Publishing Corporation.

PRINTED IN THE UNITED STATES OF AMERICA

10 9 8 7 6 5 4 3 2 1

◇ For Joshua ◇

Acknowledgments

There are many people to thank for their help, encouragement, and recipes for this book. They include Carol Jacobanis; Michael Frank; Dakota Prosch; Deborah Donenfeld; Jane Ferber; vegan and vegetarian chef Jeanette Maier; Adam Ruderman; Dr. Arthur Lebowitz; the North American Vegetarian Society; Lorna J. Sass, Ph.D.; Jennie O. Collura; Lena and Marc Romanoff; the staff at the Vegetarian Education Network; all the teenagers who offered their stories and all the health professionals who gave their advice; Joshua Ferber for his nutritional expertise; and Josh Lebowitz for his time and extraordinary editing talents. A special thanks also to Gideon Lebowitz for being so patient.

Tell me what you eat,
and I will tell you what you are.

Anthelme Brillat-Savarin, French lawyer,
economist, and author of *The Physiology
of Taste*

CONTENTS

INTRODUCTION

Nothing will benefit human health and increase the chances for survival of life on earth as much as the evolution to a vegetarian diet.

—Albert Einstein

PERHAPS nothing is more challenging in life than making a change for the better. Once you have established a pattern, altering that pattern takes hard work, perseverance, and a willingness to answer all manner of questions. If you have decided that vegetarianism is something you would like to explore and embrace, congratulations! You have begun a lifelong journey that will benefit not only your personal health immensely, but also the condition of the world in which you live.

When you first begin to investigate a vegetarian lifestyle, you may be overwhelmed by all the information and options before you. A good point to remember as you sift through information is that every aspect of vegetarianism is connected. In fact, if I could use one word to describe my vegetarian philosophy, it would be *interconnectedness*. I like the classic image of a chain, each link locked inextricably to its left and right partners.

People become vegetarians for many different reasons, but whatever the deciding factor, one step relates to another. For example, one of Mike Ravitz's motivations when he chose not to eat meat was the history of heart disease in his family. Elana Adams has raised animals all her life and cannot imagine eating one of her "friends" for dinner. Mike and

Elana have chosen to omit meat from their diets for different concerns, but their individual reasons resonate with all the issues related to vegetarianism, whether that choice is for ethical, health-related, environmental, or economic reasons.

As a teenager, I became a very strict vegetarian, refusing to eat any red meat, chicken, fish, or dairy products. I spent one summer in France eating vegetables, fruit, and bread, never once wishing that I could try a piece of *fromage* or *viande*. Another summer, while kayaking in Alaska, I never tried any of the fresh salmon that so many others were enjoying. Some people wondered whether it was difficult to resist such culinary temptations. The truth is that once you have made up your mind to do something like becoming a vegetarian, you usually do not feel deprived. Thankfully, the teens who are choosing vegetarianism today do not have quite the same hurdles that earlier vegetarians had when they stopped eating meat.

I did not know other vegetarian teens at my high school and in college, but can you imagine how lonely the Greek philosopher Pythagoras and the artist Leonardo da Vinci felt when they proclaimed that killing animals for food was cruel? The history of vegetarianism is long and varied, providing rich information from some of the world's greatest minds as to why a vegetarian lifestyle benefits not only individuals but everyone.

In the first chapter of this book, we will look at some significant vegetarians throughout history and how their efforts through the centuries have contributed to our understanding of vegetarian principles today. Knowing that so many famous people have chosen vegetarianism gives the movement a strong base and lasting credibility. Well-known historical vegetarians include Indian peace activist Mahatma Gandhi and playwright George Bernard Shaw. Today the list of celebrity vegetarians includes Natalie Merchant, Mick Jagger, Elton John, Peter Falk, Sara Gilbert, and Dustin Hoffman, to name a few.

It is important for you as a beginning vegetarian to realize that you are not alone. As overwhelmed as you feel, there are in fact untold resources, as well as a great deal of support, available to you. From magazines to youth organizations, Internet forums to local support groups, there is no reason for anyone to be alone in today's vegetarian movement. I strongly encourage people considering vegetarianism to avail themselves of the information at the back of this book before they leap into total or even partial vegetarianism. Education and awareness are your best tools when making dietary changes.

Educating yourself about vegetarianism means, among other things, learning why people become vegetarians. The reasons are as varied and specific as vegetarians themselves. In Chapter 2, we will look at why teens and others choose a meatless, and sometimes an even more austere, diet. The realities of today's livestock industry, the state of our environment, world hunger, and the gross economic inequalities that meat-for-food production promotes are not pleasant ones. To understand all the mechanisms of the meat industry, it is necessary to know how animals end up on our plates.

While researching this book, I was pleased to discover that most teens are motivated to become vegetarians after careful consideration and for a host of reasons. Many adults think that teens are not particularly concerned about their health. While a good number of the teens I spoke with chose vegetarianism for ethical reasons, many were interestesd in the health benefits as well. Some chose a vegetarian diet *solely* based on health considerations, surprising both parents and teachers alike. This is a very positive sign, considering that what teens eat today certainly affects their bodies of tomorrow.

The test results are in and they prove that high cholesterol levels, the kind that eventually lead to heart attacks and strokes, can begin in childhood. Dr. Charles R. Attwood, author of *Dr. Attwood's Low-Fat Prescription for Kids,* states, "The American Heart Association estimated in 1993 that 36 percent of American children, ages 19 and under, had high blood-cholesterol levels."[1] This means that the high level of fat consumed by most children and teens in the United States can lead to serious health problems later in life. The sooner you start on your vegetarian (and ideally low-fat) diet, the sooner you will begin on the path to a healthy future.

Today more and more teens, along with other people of all ages, are choosing a meatless diet. Some go further, giving up dairy and any other products that involve killing or using animal parts for human use. As you begin to uncover more about vegetarianism, you may wonder: Is there only one type of vegetarian? Chapter 3 looks into the different categories of vegetarians, why some people call themselves *lacto-ovo-vegetarians* and others use the term *vegan,* and whether a person can be a "partial" vegetarian. You will soon discover, once again, that the vegetarian theme has many variations.

One thing you will definitely encounter in the vegetarian world is lots of debate over what makes a true vegetarian. Each person's dietary needs are specific to him or her, just as each person's views about what to eat are different. Before you make any decisions about what degree of vegetarianism you want to commit to, explore the various options. Keep in mind that with more than 15 million North Americans calling themselves vegetarians, you are in good company.

Whatever you choose, becoming a vegetarian will change your life, and that includes relationships with parents and peers. In Chapter 4, we will focus on how to be a vegetarian and get along with family and friends. Keep in mind that any dietary alterations you make, no matter how ethical, healthy, and positive, will no doubt probably upset Mom and Dad if they are not vegetarians themselves. In fact, so many teenagers had become vegetarians by 1979 that *Time* magazine offered parents advice on how to deal with their "difficult" teens.

Parents have an enormous amount to deal with on a day-to-day basis, between working, paying bills, and raising families. News that one member of the family, and possibly more, are changing what they eat can at first trigger frustration and resentment. Eighteen-year-old Marianne Rackliffe relates that when she became a vegetarian, "My parents found the whole thing amusing. When I finally did give up all meat they thought it was 'just a phase.' Well, they were wrong."[2]

Peers and friends can also apply as much pressure as parents when one of the gang suddenly decides to stop eating meat. The teasing and questions that often ensue are exactly why educating yourself and sticking to your convictions are so important. Eliciting the help of support groups, such as Students for the Ethical Treatment of Animals (SETA) and the Vegetarian Education Network (VEN), is vital when you feel persecuted and confused. Fortunately, as more and more teens are choosing a vegetarian diet, they are finding increasing support and understanding from their peers. Schools are even heeding the call by instituting lunch programs that fit the needs of their progressively healthy student body.

You cannot be a healthy vegetarian unless you learn something about food, food groups, and basic nutrition. One thing you pick up quickly when exploring vegetarian options is that you cannot eliminate one whole food group from your diet without replacing it with an alternative to provide the nutrients you need. For fast-growing vegetarian teenagers, these can include protein, calcium, zinc, iron, and a host of other necessary nutrients. In Chapter 5, I offer comprehensive information on how you can be a nutritionally smart vegetarian while having fun in the kitchen and at the table.

One way to learn about the new foods you will encounter is to cook with them. Even if you have never boiled a potato, there is no reason why you cannot step into the kitchen and take charge of your meals. You are probably thinking, "When do I have time to cook between band rehearsal, softball practice, the school play, and homework?" I have compiled recipes in Chapter 6 with an active teen schedule in mind, and with the understanding that for adolescents, food is often eaten on the run. You will learn to make such simple delicacies as English muffin pizzas, tacos, veggie burgers, baked apples, and trail mix, among other delicious foods.

As I mentioned before, the back of the book is full of current and important information for anyone looking into vegetarianism. Groups, books, magazines, Internet forums, and other sources for material are all accessible by simple phone calls, a walk to the bookstore or library, or using a modem. You will discover literally millions of other vegetarians in the United States and around the world, once you begin to search for them.

Next to infancy, you experience your fastest rate of growth during adolescence. As a result, it is vital that you maintain a healthy diet to accommodate your body's ever-changing nutritional needs. Parents, doctors, and nutritionists may tell you that vegetarianism is just not safe for a blossoming teen. Fortunately, you can dispel this myth simply by informing yourself of the facts. This book and others help explain how vegetarianism is healthy not only for adults, but also for teens and even infants. You are going through all sorts of changes now, physical and otherwise. Asserting your independence is very important now; overcoming difficult odds is one way to illustrate to your parents, teachers, and peers that you are well on your way to responsible adulthood.

Remember to approach each challenge of your vegetarianism with the knowledge that you are doing something profoundly positive not only for yourself, but also for the world that you will inherit. Looking to the past is one of the best ways to learn how to navigate the future; in the first chapter of this book, we will look at the history of vegetarianism and its development through the ages.

PART ONE

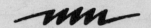

HOW IT ALL BEGAN:
The History of Vegetarianism

1

STANDING THE TEST OF TIME

I have from an early age abjured the use of meat, and the time will come when men such as I will look on the murder of animals as they now look on the murder of men.

—Leonardo da Vinci

VEGETARIANISM has been around for a long, long time. No one is sure exactly how long, but there is evidence that since prehistoric times, the human diet has consisted mostly of plant foods. We will take a journey starting near the beginning of recorded time all the way up to the present era to discover the very roots of the vegetarian diet. It is a fascinating trip, filled with stories and legends about famous writers, artists, painters, philosophers, and musicians. You will easily recognize some names, while others may be new to you. Imagine how your skeptical parents will react when you tell them that the vegetarian company you keep includes the Greek philosopher Pythagoras; writers Leo Tolstoy and Isaac Bashevis Singer; one of the greatest triathletes of all time, Dave Scott; and rock singers Michael Stipe and Natalie Merchant, among others.

IN THE BEGINNING THERE WAS SOME MEAT

IN PREHISTORIC TIMES, people moved around a lot. Tribes led nomadic lives, never staying in one place too long, because they had to base their diets on the seasons and the move-

3

ments of animals. Early humans, including Neanderthals and Cro-Magnons, no doubt ate some flesh, but they also mixed many plant foods into their diets.

We will never know many animals were hunted, killed, and eaten; however, anthropology, the study of groups and societies of people, can dispel certain myths about our early relatives. According to Virginia and Mark Messina, co-authors of *The Vegetarian Way,* "Our earliest ancestors probably didn't hunt animals. Rather, they scavenged, eating the meager leftovers at the kill site after other animals had feasted and left."[1] Early humans did do some hunting and scavenging, but they were probably not the mighty hunters that we have been led to believe.

NO DAIRY IN THOSE DAYS

DIETS IN PREHISTORIC times revolved around what vegetables, fruits, nuts, seeds, and meat our ancestors could find. People were unable to digest dairy—and there were no domesticated cows to offer them milk anyway. Despite the fact that early humans did not consume dairy products, they had a very high intake of calcium. One explanation for this centers on their high consumption of wild greens, which were rich in calcium.

We know that groups of people in prehistoric times had adequate calcium supplies because their bones were so massive. We will learn more about why calcium is so important in our diets in Chapter 5.

WE START TO SETTLE DOWN

WHEN THE FIRST agricultural systems appeared sometime between 10,000 and 12,000 years ago, humans started to settle down into communities and began growing crops of plant foods.

Once vegetables and fruits became dominant in the diet, meat became less of a mainstay in their meals. People did not entirely give up eating animals, but instead of scavenging them, they now raised them as livestock. Eating meat gradually became part of a more advanced system of cultivating food, also based on a seasonal calendar for ceremonial purposes and in times of need when other food was scarce. As time passed, meat consumption became more of a luxury than an actual need, as communities realized that they could survive on plant foods alone.

As agricultural communities grew, the seeds of civilization were sown, and groups began preparing food for pleasure. Early chefs developed new ways to combine and cook food, laying the groundwork for a long tradition of culinary arts in different and emerging cultures. As you can imagine, cuisines of developing societies depended on whatever resources were available to them as well as when these foods were in season.

From these agricultural communities sprang kingdoms, villages, towns, and eventually cities. With the advent of civilization, people realized that having more land, animals, and possessions made you more powerful than your neighbor. Certain families rose to the highest tier of society and became royalty. There were definitely hierarchical divisions and inequalities between the prehistoric tribes, but people became much more organized about power once they stopped having to move around all the time.

As people began to divide into classes of rich and poor, society often measured their wealth, or lack of it, by how much livestock they had. In other words, raising animals for meat became a status symbol, one that poorer people could not afford. In the Bible, King Solomon provided lavish dinners of meat for his guests, and biblical society measured the wealth and status of other patriarchs by how many cattle, sheep, and goats they owned. During modern times, the same societal convention has held true. Those cultures that are prosperous tend to eat meat as a show of their wealth. However, many of the world's most nutritionally healthy cultures have almost always been vegetarian, like China. Chinese society has almost always survived on a simple vegetarian diet, especially the historically large peasant class. Rice and bean curd (tofu) appear in Chinese literature as symbols of the poor, but they have also come to suggest a life of simplicity and virtue. While royalty in China feasted throughout the ages upon such meat dishes as fried snake relish and quail sautéed with bamboo shoots, the peasant's more austere fare has been the mainstay of the Chinese diet for centuries.

Interestingly, the Chinese diet based on grains, vegetables, and soy products is one of the healthiest in the world. The Chinese who maintain the traditional diet have some of the lowest incidence of heart disease and cancer on the planet. In Chapter 5 we will discuss why a diet consisting largely of grains and vegetables is by far the healthiest no matter where you live.

GREECE

THE MAN CONSIDERED the "father" of vegetarianism was a sixth-century-B.C. Greek philosopher named Pythagoras. Pythagoras, born in approximately 580 B.C., was also a brilliant mathematician and theorist, and is perhaps best known as the discoverer of the Pythagorean theorem and many other mathematical ideas. He believed that the earth moved around the sun, something not yet proven in his day, and founded a society that thought meat-eating was taboo. He contended that a vegetarian lifestyle was the most natural and healthiest around. In fact, it is believed that, thanks to Pythagoras, the "real" vegetarian movement started in ancient Greece.

Pythagoras was able to convince many other important Greek philosophers, including Socrates and Plato, that vegetarianism was the best way to eat. Many future vegetarians, including George Bernard Shaw and Dr. J. H. Kellogg, were greatly influenced by the progressive Greek philosopher. In fact, the term *vegetarianism* was not used to describe non–meat eaters until the late nineteenth century. Until that time, people on a meatless diet were called *Pythagoreans*.

ROME

DESPITE THE FACT that the Romans fashioned an unusually aggressive society, their armies conquered most of the known world on a vegetarian diet. A Roman soldier's meal generally consisted of bread, porridge, vegetables, wine, and occasionally fish. According to historian Will Durant, when Roman troops ran out of corn, they were upset at having to eat meat.[2]

Throughout history, it has been the rich who ate meat because they could afford it, and ancient Rome was no exception. Wealthy citizens of Rome enjoyed not just their own domesticated breeds of animals, but also the flesh of exotic animals, such as peacocks. It was the army and the proletariat, or lower classes, who enjoyed the benefits of a vegetarian diet.

Leonardo da Vinci (1452–1519)

After the decline of the Roman Empire, around the middle of the fifth century A.D., the vegetarian diet generally fell out of favor. Of course there were some vegetarians between the fifth century and the nineteenth century, when vegetarianism became popular again. One of the most notable vegetarians during this period was the Italian artist Leonardo da Vinci.

Da Vinci loved animals. He was very fond of horses and liked to buy birds from merchants in order to release them. He believed the killing of animals for food to be cruel and inhumane. In his notebook, referring to sheep, cows, goats, and other livestock animals, he wrote, "Endless number of these animals shall have their little children taken from them, ripped open, and barbarously slaughtered." And of boiled fish, he wrote, "How cruel for one whose natural habitat is water to be made to die in boiling water."[3]

Clearly Leonardo da Vinci was a vegetarian for ethical reasons. His notebooks are filled with entries bemoaning the plight of animals used for human consumption. Not only did he not eat meat, but he also condemned the use of cheese, eggs, and honey, leading us to believe that he was also a vegan.

A Popular Movement Is Born

After the fifth century and before the nineteenth, the best-known groups practicing vegetarianism in Europe were a few orders of the Catholic Church, such as the Benedictines and the Cistercians. Individually, such historical luminaries as William Shakespeare and Benjamin Franklin chose a meatless diet. However, it was not until the nineteenth century that the "modern" vegetarian movement really got under way.

The first vegetarian movement was started largely by people in England and the United States known as "diet reformers." These were nutrition experts who believed that a diet consisting of meat, among other things, corrupted the body. They believed people should regard their bodies as temples, as the ancient Greeks had. There were various colorful characters in the early modern vegetarian movement, many of whom attracted large groups of followers in search of a purer way of life.

THE FIRST OF MANY

THE BIBLE CHRISTIANS, a group of English people who tried to live their lives according to what they believed were strict biblical principles, founded the Vegetarian Society of Great Britain in 1847. This society was the first of its kind; its founders probably had no idea how many more societies would follow its lead. The British society coined the term *vegetarian,* which derives from the Latin word *vegetare*, meaning "enliven." As mentioned before, vegetarians before this time had called themselves *Pythagoreans*.

Fueled by an interest in good health and kindness to animals, members of vegetarian societies began to meet for discussion and support. It was not difficult for people to become vegetarians because in reality most people in Europe and the United States during the nineteenth century could not afford much meat anyway.

GEORGE BERNARD SHAW (1856–1950)

GEORGE BERNARD SHAW, the author of such plays as *Candida* and *Pygmalion*, was a devout vegetarian for well over half his life. The Englishman wrote numerous magazine articles and letters declaring his passionate belief that killing animals for human consumption was nothing short of evil. Shaw was one of the few vegetarians in his circle; people were always trying to convince him that his diet was unhealthy—even his doctor. One medical professional even ascribed a boil on Shaw's cheek to his vegetarianism.

Shaw never relented in his commitment to a meatless diet and was a dedicated vegetarian for decades. The playwright believed that " . . . persons who have never from their birth been . . . otherwise than as vegetarians are at no disadvantage, mentally, physically, nor in duration of life."[4] Shaw himself lived to the ripe old age of 94.

COMING TO AMERICA

BIBLE CHRISTIAN MINISTER William Metcalf left England in 1817 with 41 church members and brought vegetarianism across the Atlantic Ocean to the United States. While Metcalf and his congregation declared the benefits of a vegetarian diet, other American religious leaders, such as John and Charles Wesley, the founders of Methodism, also promoted the healthful aspects of vegetarianism.

In response to the establishment of the Vegetarian Society of Great Britain in 1847, Metcalf encouraged diet reformers in the United States to create an American counterpart. In 1850, the American Vegetarian Society held its first convention. The vegetarian cause in the United States was also taken up by the nineteenth-century doctor Anna Kingsford. She stated that some of the strongest animals in the world, such as horses, camels, and elephants, subsisted only on plants. They did not need meat or dairy products to make them physically powerful.

People began to experiment with healthier lifestyles, which included vegetarianism. In the United States, groups formed to promote a more natural and basic way of life. One such venture in vegetarian living was called Fruitlands.

FRUITLANDS

THE FRUITLANDS COMMUNITY, founded in Harvard, Massachusetts, in 1843 by Charles Lane and Amos Bronson Alcott, espoused all the values of the vegan diet. The fare at Fruitlands consisted of fruit, grains, beans, and peas. The members of the commune shunned meat, fish, butter, cheese, eggs, and milk because they felt that animal products corrupted the body.

The Fruitlands community also believed in goodwill toward their fellow humans, not just animals. They refused to use tea, coffee, rice, molasses, and sugar because slaves were used to produce these items.

Unfortunately, the community only lasted seven months because the group was not particularly productive. Most members spent their time sitting around discussing lofty ideas rather than growing the food they needed. Amos Bronson Alcott's daughter Louisa, author of *Little Women*, wrote a satire about Fruitlands in *Transcendental Wild Oats*.

SEVENTH-DAY ADVENTISTS

OFTEN CREDITED WITH being one of the most important influences on the American vegetarian movement, the Seventh-Day Adventists have been teaching the ways of vegetarianism since the mid-nineteenth century. Ellen White, who founded the church in 1840, wrote extensively on the importance of spiritual and physical health. She was not only a great proponent of a healthy diet and exercise, but also a supporter of John Harvey Kellogg. In fact, White and her husband, James, hired Kellogg as a doctor at their Western Health Reform Institute in Battle Creek, Michigan. Kellogg later named it the Battle Creek Sanitarium.

Today members of the church are among the most active in promoting vegetarianism, with nearly all of the clergy abstaining from meat. Seventh-Day Adventists have always been interested in getting the word out and have many community outreach programs that focus on diet and health. They also own several food companies and restaurants that sell vegetarian products and food.

BATTLE CREEK SANITARIUM

JOHN HARVEY KELLOGG, the man who invented cornflakes, was a fanatical diet reformer in the late nineteenth century. Kellogg ran a sanitarium in Battle Creek, Michigan, where he tried to create the healthiest environment possible. He and his wife developed tasty vegetarian foods for their clients, spending many hours in the kitchen experimenting with different recipes. He invented several types of food, including meat analogues (foods that replace meat in the diet with the same nutrients) and peanut butter.

Kellogg encouraged his patients to give up not only meat, but other foods that he thought were harmful, including chocolate and alcohol. Kellogg was a perfect example of someone who led a healthy vegetarian lifestyle, including plenty of physical activity in his daily routine. He lived to the age of 91.

WORLD WAR I (1914–1918)

VEGETARIANISM GAINED A scientific base during World War I, when citizens in the United States and Europe had to omit meat from their diets due to a scarcity of food. Scientists in the United States were afforded a unique look at how a diet without meat affected the population. While investigating alternatives to meat and protein, they discovered the benefits of a vegetarian lifestyle. Scientists noticed an overall improvement in health and a lower mortality rate. Naturally, when the war ended and people resumed eating meat, overall health declined and the mortality rate increased again. Not surprisingly, the same phenomenon occurred during World War II in the 1940s.

MEAT AND DAIRY TAKE HOLD

IN THE EARLY 1940s, the estimated number of vegetarians living in the United States was 2.5 to 3 million, which was about 2 percent of the population. After World War II ended in 1945, the United States government began distributing guides that promoted both meat and dairy for good health. Meat and dairy products were symbols of a country that had finished struggling with war and was ready for better times and richer diets. As a result, both the meat and dairy industries became very powerful with the help of the government and have since tried to maintain their stronghold on our diets. I'm sure many of your parents, and perhaps you too, can remember material handed out in school that stressed the importance of beef, chicken, fish, eggs, and milk in our daily diet.

VEGETARIANISM ON THE RISE

DURING THE 1950s, more Americans were eating meat and dairy products than ever before. It was not until the late 1960s and 1970s that vegetarianism experienced a renaissance, or rebirth. The 1960s saw the rise of counterculture groups in the United States—groups that protested against the Vietnam War, the government, parental authority, and destruction of the environment. People who were involved in the "back-to-nature" and peace movements were interested in a healthier way of life, and this included vegetarianism. Many gave up meat because it was better for them and the planet. They also stopped eating meat for ethical reasons and out of concern for animals.

Frances Moore Lappé's *Diet for a Small Planet,* published in 1971, is often cited as one of the most important books promoting vegetarianism. She discusses how a vegetarian diet is not only healthy for individuals, but also for the environment. She also argues that if people eat less meat, there is more land to grow food for people instead of livestock.

VEGETARIANISM FOR THE FUTURE

THE ANIMAL RIGHTS movement continued to grow during the 1970s and 1980s with the publication of Peter Singer's

Animal Liberation and the formation of the group People for the Ethical Treatment of Animals (PETA). The medical community also presented its facts on how eating meat is plainly bad for your health. In fact, the Physicians Committee for Responsible Medicine promotes a vegetarian diet above all others.

Today, vegetarianism is moving closer and closer to the American mainstream, with restaurants, convenience stores, supermarkets, and health food stores supplying tasty and healthy meat alternatives. Anyone choosing vegetarianism today is in good company. The list of celebrities, athletes, artists, and politicians embracing the cause grows each year, with books, magazines, and Internet groups all providing a strong base of support.

STRENGTH IN NUMBERS

AS THE LEGIONS of vegetarians grow, so too does their power. More than 12 million Americans consider themselves vegetarians, which is about 5 percent of the population. According to a poll taken by *Vegetarian Times* magazine, the number of vegetarians increased 33 percent between 1985 and 1992. Another survey by Teenage Research Unlimited found that 33 percent of teenage girls and 17 percent of teenage boys think vegetarianism is "in." Soon supermarkets and fast-food restaurants such as McDonald's will have to offer alternatives to meat and dairy or they will lose business. As more and more teenagers become vegetarians, they will begin to change the way their world eats by making their preferences known.

In Chapter 2, we will answer the question that almost every vegetarian is asked: Why did you choose vegetarianism? As you will see, the replies are as diverse as the individuals who become vegetarians.

PART TWO

━━〰〰〰━━

WHAT'S IT ALL ABOUT:
Vegetarianism in Our Lives

— 2 —

THE VEGETARIAN LIFE FOR ME

My refusing to eat flesh occasioned an inconvenience, and
I was frequently chided for my singularity, but with this
lighter repast I made the greater progress, from greater clearness
of head and quicker comprehension.

—Benjamin Franklin

YOU have announced to your family and friends that you
are no longer eating meat and they all want to know why.
Hopefully, if you are telling people that you are embracing
vegetarianism, in whatever form, you have spent some time
thinking the matter over. Sally Clinton, founder of the
Vegetarian Education Network (VEN), believes more teens
are becoming vegetarians because "there is more information, so there's more awareness." If you educate yourself
about vegetarianism, you will discover the myriad of reasons why people choose a meatless diet. They include:

◇ Ethics
◇ Health
◇ Environment
◇ Economics
◇ Religion
◇ No taste for meat
◇ Media influence
◇ Peer pressure
◇ Teenage rebellion

◈Vegetarian parents

◈Eating disorders

It is true that some teens simply decide they are no longer eating meat, and they do not have any strong convictions about the matter. Generally, however, teens who do become vegetarians have given the subject a great deal of consideration; as 15-year-old Heather Mandel says, "I guess kids my age are just questioning the world." Aware of the facts and their feelings, teens are ready to answer the first question their parents, teachers, and peers usually pose to them: Why?

Ethics

MOST TEENAGERS SAY they become vegetarians for ethical reasons. This means that they believe that killing animals for food is wrong. Many teens who choose vegetarianism are shocked when they learn how the animals people consume are treated during their often too-brief lives. Most teens are unaware of the patently inhumane practices of the meat and dairy industries. The gross mistreatment of animals on their way to being a Big Mac or veal scallopini further strengthens a new vegetarian's conviction that he or she has made the right choice.

How Can I Eat My Friends?

Most children grow up inundated with images of animals. When they are babies, friends and relatives offer stuffed rabbits, lambs, and baby chicks to welcome an infant into the world. As they grow, children's books, television shows, and movies convey the message that animals are among their closest friends. Marcie Welsh, 16, remembers, "At the time I wasn't exactly sure why I became a vegetarian, but I always saw animals personified on TV, and I had this image of Bessie the cow being slaughtered and put on my plate. I thought, what if she ate me?"

Additionally, if a family considers bringing a pet into their home, they usually do so when children are young. A child learns much from taking care of another life, understanding that taking responsibility for an animal is hard work, but that it is also endlessly rewarding. For many teens, pets are among their closest companions. Elana Adams says, "We moved around a lot when I was young and our dog Tarzan was sometimes my only friend."

Now imagine you are one day out in the yard playing with your pet baby chicks and the next thing you know, you are at the dinner table about to dine on roasted chicken. For a lot of people the link between the living animals and the ones on the plate is never made. Not so for 17-year-old Mike Ravitz, who began making the connection when his father brought home some baby chicks for him:

My father is a doctor and at one point, he worked in a wheelchair community. The people who worked at the community hatched baby chicks for the residents. One day, my father was walking by a box and saw some fluffy chickens. He took two chicks home for me and my brother. From then on, I took care of the chickens. One evening, I had just come inside from playing with the chicks and sat down to dinner. There was a chicken on my plate and I said, "This isn't right, I can't eat this." Right then and there, I told my parents that I wasn't eating any more meat. Over time, I started to learn more about the decision I had made. I talked to people, I attended programs, and I learned more about vegetarianism. I learned that it made sense. I became a strict vegetarian about three years ago, a vegan. It all goes back to the little box of fluffy chickens.

EATING ANIMALS IS WRONG

Newsweek recently reported that "[c]oncern for animals is the leading reason why kids give up eating meat."[1]

College student Claire Adams agrees when she states, "I find it incomprehensible that people kill animals to eat them." For her, taking the life of another creature for dietary purposes is unacceptable and unjust. Like Claire, many teens think that eating animals is just plain cruel. According to artist Sue Coe, author of *Dead Meat*, "Animals have the right not to end up on the ends of our forks." As you read in the previous chapter, many famous historical figures refrained from eating meat out of their compassion for animals. *Rights* and *compassion*: Teens often use these two words when they describe their attitude toward animals.

As more teens become vegetarians, they are conveying the message that they want a more peaceful, less violent world by attempting to stop the slaughter of so many animals for food. In the United States alone, over 7 billion animals are killed for food each year, not including fish.

LOVE FOR ANIMALS

As we discussed earlier, children often learn to love by caring for animals.

Their first attachments are often to the family dog, a pony at a local stable, or a cow at a farm in the country. Elana Adams, who is now 20 and became a vegetarian when she was 10, tells why she chose to stop eating meat:

I grew up surrounded by animals and really loved them. I didn't really make the connection between eating meat and animals until I . . . saw a pig slaughtered. I was very disturbed by that and just kept thinking about it. That day was the first time I really associated meat with the suffering of an animal. I stopped eating red meat first, but still ate chicken and fish. About a year later, I was at my uncle's house and they had all these little ducks and that's when I stopped eating fowl. A year after that in Norway, we were eating salmon with a group of environmentalists and they were talking about the salmon migration and eating it at the same time. That's when I stopped eating fish. I gave things up slowly which probably made it easier. I certainly don't miss meat anymore.

Elana, like many of her vegetarian peers, feels that the life of an animal is just as important as that of a human being and, as such, is one that deserves respect.

FACTORY FARMING

Many teens give up meat because they think killing animals for food is fundamentally wrong.

As Sally Clinton of the Vegetarian Education Network (VEN) says, "When they realize that meat is a dead animal, that's reason enough for a lot of kids to stop eating it."[2] What many kids are not aware of is how most food animals actually live before they end up in the grocery store or at the butcher.

Raising livestock that eventually become hamburgers, pork chops, and chicken wings is very big business. Gone are the days of the small family farm, where cows, pigs, and chickens roamed the fields and barnyards mooing, oinking, and clucking their days away. Today, large factory farms raise animals for food. The owners of these factories are not interested in the welfare of these creatures, but in how much money they can make from them in the shortest amount of time.

In factory farms, animals are treated like machines, not living, breathing beings. Most of these factories are:

◇ *Dark:* Animals need light, just as we do, so they know when to go to bed and when to be awake. In the murky darkness of most factory farms and slaughterhouses, animals lose touch with their own natural cycles and habits because their sense of time and place is lost. How can a hen rise with the sun when she never sees it?

◇ *Poorly ventilated:* The factories are large and have poor air circulation. Animals are often so crowded together that some suffocate. In winter, the air is cold because it costs too much to heat. In summer, the reverse is true and temperatures rise to unbearable heights. Animals go crazy from the heat and are rarely given enough water or space to keep hydrated and cool.

◇ *Overcrowded:* Space is very important to animals. They need it, just as we do, to move around, stretch, and feel comfortable. Factory farms do not allow animals nearly enough space to keep them healthy. The owners of the farms think the more animals they can cram into one space, the more meat they will produce, and the more money they will make. Many creatures die due to the close conditions under which they live, but the owners figure these losses into their profits.

◇*Full of disease:* Because of the first three reasons listed here, and others, many animals
become very sick. There is no time to take care
of these ailing creatures so most of them are
killed or simply left to die. To keep large
amounts of animals from getting sick, factory
farms administer enormous doses of antibiotics
(medicines that fight bacterial infections and
diseases) to the animals. This keeps some of
them alive longer, but it ultimately does not
solve the problem; the drugs end up in the meat
we eat and the milk we drink.

One visit to a factory farm or a slaughterhouse and most
people would instantly become vegetarians. The conditions
under which individual animals live and how they are
treated is extremely disturbing, but very important to know
if you are choosing vegetarianism for ethical reasons.

COWS

Where the cow is kept and cared for, Civilization advances, land grows
richer, homes grow better, debts grow fewer.

—Paul Hamilton Hayne, nineteenth century
American poet

Take a moment and think about cows. What ideas and images
come to mind? Probably you imagine a rather docile, not
very intelligent, somewhat peaceful creature. While cows are
gentle, they are by no means dumb or unaware. In fact, a
mother cow can identify her own calf in a herd of hundreds
of other baby cows. Cows are playful and sensitive, and they
love to walk through fields, searching for the sweetest clover
and grasses to munch on. Most of us imagine cows in a red

barn surrounded by other content farm animals.

Unfortunately, in today's meat and dairy markets, cows are not able to amble lazily in fields of delicious greens.

HAMBURGER LOTS: You may think that most beef cattle, the kind that become steaks and hamburgers, roam the open range grazing and chewing until it is time for them to be slaughtered. But, in fact, by the early part of the 1970s, three-quarters of U.S. beef cattle were living their lives in feedlots. These dirty, overcrowded lots, where cattle are often fed newspaper, cement, and their own excrement, are their last homes before they are killed.

In order to get to these feedlots, cattle are jammed into crowded and foul-smelling trucks that are freezing cold in winter and stiflingly hot in summer. Many go crazy from the overcrowding and smell, collapse, and are trampled by other cattle.

Scores of animals die in transit, yet rather than improve the system, beef companies just write them off as a loss. Once at the feedlots, the cattle are often castrated to produce a higher percentage of body fat and thus more meat. They are then dehorned when and if they go berserk from the stress; without horns, they will not damage other animals. Next comes branding with a hot iron, and then finally a dose of hormones, antibiotics, and chemicals. The drugs and chemicals cause the animals to gain weight faster, become more resistant to disease, and hopefully survive under the gross conditions of the feedlot until it is time for slaughter.

THE MILK FACTORY: In milk factories, cows are essentially four-legged machines with one purpose: to produce as much milk as possible. In order to do this, each cow must be pregnant almost all the time. Milk cows are given hormones so that they can easily become pregnant and make more milk. But cows are not meant to be perpetually having babies. Doing so puts enormous wear on their bodies. In addition, the hormones make a cow's udder so unnaturally full of milk that even if her calves were allowed to suckle, they would probably hurt it. Normally, cows have a life expectancy of 20 to 25 years, but under the stressful conditions in the milk factory, most make it only to about age 4.

Milk cows are not allowed to wander around, but instead are kept in dark concrete stalls with slatted metal floors. The cow is overly tense from always being pregnant, nervous because she never gets to move around, and upset because her babies are taken away from her as soon as they are born. This "most mellow and patient of animals"[3] is now a jittery mess and is often given tranquilizers to calm her down.

Chained around the neck in her stall with an electric pumping machine hooked up to her udder, it is no surprise that the modern milk cow does not survive very long in the factory.

THE TRAGEDY OF VEAL: Veal has gained a tragically special place in the nefarious saga of the cattle industry. Veal comes from the male offspring of milk cows; their meat has long been regarded as a gourmet food. Since the horrors of veal production have been revealed to the general public, more and more people are refusing to eat it, and more and more restaurants will no longer serve it.

Veal calves are separated from their mothers only two or three days after birth and placed in crates so small that they cannot stand up. They are housed with other calves or alone; they are rarely alone in their natural environment. Calves are playful by nature; when not suckling from or being licked by their mothers, they generally like to frolic and run with the herd.

Veal calves are not allowed to move because that would cause them to develop muscles, which would make their meat tough and undesirable to gourmands. Consigned to their uncomfortable crates for their entire lives, the calves are fed on a diet of milk that is very low in iron and makes them anemic. Again, this is so their flesh will be pale and tender when it is time for slaughter.

Calves have a very strong sucking reflex, like most babies, so they can drink their mother's milk. A veal calf will desperately try to suck anything, but he is often muzzled so he cannot get any extra iron from the metal on his harness or the bars of his stall. Calves are almost always kept in wooden crates to avoid the possibility of getting any extra iron from the bars on a metal cage.

Recently, thanks to the growing awareness of the inhumane practices concerning veal, a large-scale campaign has been waged, to make life better for these creatures. Unfortunately, an organization called The National Grange, which dedicates itself to the advancement of agriculture, has blocked any serious reform.

You can help the campaign against veal by becoming a member of an animal rights group, such as the People for the Ethical Treatment of Animals (PETA), and letting your voice be heard.

PIGS

The commonly held image of pigs as greedy, fat, and filthy creatures, gross beasts who eat anything that isn't fastened down, and who selfishly indulge their basest instincts without a trace of sensitivity, could hardly be further from the truth.

—John Robbins, activist and author of
Diet for a New America

There is no doubt that pigs have a bad reputation for being slovenly, lazy, and not good for much except pork chops and bacon. In reality, pigs are smart and clean; they roll around in the mud only because they have no sweat glands, and the mud keeps them cool. Generally, pigs love to have fun and are very sociable. It is because of the way humans tend to treat pigs that they have strayed so far from their natural behavior.

PIG FACTORIES: Today, the modern factory-housed pig is kept under conditions that make it impossible for it to stay clean. Pigs rarely live on bucolic farms anymore; instead they are usually born, raised, and slaughtered in huge industrial complexes. Pig factories often have over 100,000 animals, each kept in a stall so small that it cannot turn around or lie down. The stalls are built over slatted floors, which allow urine and feces to fall into a large pit directly below the cages. The slatted design painfully maims the cloven-hoofed foot of the pig, as the slats cut into the animal's feet.

The waste from the cages is rarely cleaned, so the odors, germs, and toxic gases rise from the pits, spreading disease. Tragically, pigs have very sensitive noses and are greatly affected by the noxious and disgusting smells surrounding them. In addition, you can imagine their misery as they stand in their crates, breathing in the foul odors with nowhere to go, no way to escape.

SAUSAGE MACHINES: Pig farmers are very excited at the prospect that their sows can now produce nearly seven times the piglets they would normally give birth to in nature. According to an article in *National Hog Farmer*, "The breeding sow should be thought of, treated as, a valuable piece of machinery, whose function is to pump out baby pigs like a sausage machine."[4] The babies are taken away from their mother almost immediately and fed by a machine.

Meanwhile, the mother pig, thanks to hormone injections, can start the process of breeding again.

As with life in cow feedlots, life in a pig factory is so stressful for the animals that many go insane and begin biting off the tails of other pigs when they are penned together. Pig producers have found a way to combat this problem by simply cutting off their pigs' tails as a preventive measure. This practice is called "tail-docking" and is a very painful procedure that generally makes the pigs even more upset and disturbed.

Not surprisingly, many pigs die under these horrendous conditions, but again the modern pork producer just figures the deaths into his total stock, price structure, and profit. The pig, a naturally sensitive and peaceful creature, is transformed into a miserable and nervous animal by an industry that views it only as a "sausage machine."

CHICKENS

> Hickety pickety, my black hen,
> She lays eggs for gentlemen.
> Gentlemen come every day
> To see what my black hen doth lay.
>
> —"Hickety Pickety," Anonymous

Confined like the cows and pigs, chickens no longer spend their days aimlessly clucking around the barnyard scratching for worms and tending to their chicks. In children's stories like "The Little Red Hen," chickens are portrayed as hardworking, industrious, and determined. In modern chicken farms, the birds no longer possess any of these qualities that are natural and instinctive to them.

OUT OF THE COOP: Hens that lay eggs (*layers*) no longer live in coops laying eggs according to the natural cycles of the day, but in chicken factories that are devoid of light, proper ventilation, and space. They live jammed five or more to a cage and are there for no other purpose but to lay as many eggs as they possibly can each day. Due to the stress of their confinement, chickens often furiously peck at one another. Similarly to the tail-docking practice with pigs and the dehorning of cows, chickens are routinely debeaked to avoid hurting each other. However, their beaks are taken off by machines that often cut painfully into their flesh and leave them vulnerable to infections and disease.

BROILERS: Chickens that are bred solely for their meat are referred to by the poultry industry as *broilers*. Chickens, which normally have a life expectancy of 15 to 20 years, usually live no longer than 2 months before they head to the grocery store or butcher. Modern chicken breeders are in search of the perfect broiler, one with a bulging breast and not much else. Chickens are fed on a diet of hormones to make their breast meat plump, but the heavy chest makes the rest of their skeleton weak. The birds are often so physically compromised after all the tampering that they need heavy doses of antibiotics to keep them free of infection before they are slaughtered.

FEET AND FEATHERS: Chickens, like pigs, also develop foot problems in their cages. In the dirt, a chicken's nails are kept naturally clipped by her scratching and walking. In the cages, where there is nowhere for the birds to move, their nails quickly become overgrown and entwined in the mesh where they continue to grow, literally strapping the chickens to their own cages.

Farmers also force chickens to molt more than they

would naturally, by withholding food and water for up to a week and a half at a time. The greater the amount of molting, the more eggs the chickens will produce. Unfortunately, birds that are not strong enough quickly die from starvation, and in fact, 3 to 4 percent of chickens die in this manner.

MALE CHICKS: Each day thousands of chicks are born in chicken factories. The females become layers like their mothers, while the males are pitched live into garbage bags and thrown away in the trash. If they are not discarded immediately, the male chicks are often crushed up and used as fertilizer in fields. Sue Coe writes in her book *Dead Meat*, "Walking along a plowed field, you can sometimes find a chick, still alive, with no legs or wings."[5]

A PLEA FOR THE ANIMALS

As you can see, the life of animals in modern factory farms is almost too horrible to imagine. Many teens, when they learn how bad the conditions are, renounce meat as a protest against the treatment of creatures intended for our sandwiches, barbecues, and dinner parties. The reason most people do not know about the practices of factory farms is because the industries like to keep their methods hidden. Imagine the outcry if everyone knew how cows, pigs, and chickens, not to mention lambs, turkeys, and fish, spent their days.

By choosing vegetarianism, teenagers are taking action against the modern food factory system, and are sending a strong message to the industry's leaders: It is time to change.

HEALTH

AS MENTIONED BEFORE, according to *Newsweek*, the main reason kids stop eating meat is "concern for animals."[6] However, many teens believe that the health benefits from a vegetarian diet are equally important. Mike Ravitz says, "I became a vegetarian for ethical reasons, but now the health and ethical reasons have become combined."

Hundreds of scientific studies clearly illustrate that a vegetarian diet is far healthier than a meat-based one and that the earlier a person stops eating meat, and in some cases dairy also, the better. Many people think that what young children or teens eat will not affect them later on in life, but this is patently untrue. What we eat when we are young has far-reaching consequences of which we are often tragically unaware until it is too late to do anything about them.

THE PROBLEMS WITH EATING MEAT AND DAIRY

You can develop many diseases when you eat a diet based largely on meat and dairy products. While it is not always easy to eliminate both these food groups from your diet, you should know the many problems they can cause. Starting slowly and gradually eliminating foods, as we will discuss in later chapters, and not just suddenly dropping foods, is the best way to begin changing your dietary habits.

Some of the health problems we will explore include:

◇ Heart/coronary artery disease

◇ Cancer

◇ High blood pressure

◇ Diabetes

◇Osteoporosis

◇Lactose intolerance

◇Obesity

and the adverse effects of:

◇Hormones

◇Antibiotics

◇Additives and Pesticides

A vegetarian diet centered on whole grains, legumes, vegetables, and fruits can help reduce the risk of all of these health problems.

HEART/CORONARY ARTERY DISEASE: Most teens are not overly concerned about having heart attacks or whether their arteries are clogged. Unfortunately, these problems *should* concern them.

◇Meat and dairy products contain a large amount of fat, specifically saturated fat, which can raise the amount of cholesterol in your blood to dangerously high levels.

◇There are two types of cholesterol: LDL and HDL. Scientists often call LDL the "bad" cholesterol and HDL the "good" cholesterol. The fat in animal products raises the levels of LDL in your blood, which is transported to your heart through the bloodstream.

◇Cholesterol, on its way to your heart, forms a thick plaque along the walls of the arteries. If these arteries clog, then less and less blood reaches your heart over the years until, eventually, you have a heart attack. Each year thousands of people in the United States die from heart attacks who never even knew they had a problem.

Since the 1960s, when the condition was the cause of over half the deaths in North America, coronary artery disease has been on the decline. This is due to advancements in medicine and to people cutting back on their fat intake and getting more exercise. Vegetables tend to contain very small amounts of fat and have no cholesterol, so a vegetarian diet is by far the healthiest for your heart.

While diet plays a significant if not primary role in keeping your heart pumping, your genes may also have a lot to do with it. People are born with genetic material that their parents have passed on to them. Some families have a greater disposition to high levels of blood cholesterol than others. If you know that your grandfather and your mother both have to keep an eye on their cholesterol levels, chances are that you should too. Have your doctor do some tests to find out how high your cholesterol is and make your decisions based on the results.

You may decide, as Mike Ravitz did, that a vegetarian diet is the best way to stay healthy. He relates:

The health benefits of vegetarianism are very important to me. My grandfather was a meatpacker. He had a prosperous meatpacking plant in Nebraska and became quite rich. I never met him because he died of a heart attack. My father inherited the genetic tendency for heart disease. Two years ago, my father had bypass surgery to prevent his arteries from becoming too clogged. He chose to prevent a heart attack. He woke up to the fact that having a steak every day was harmful to his health. He now eats a very healthy vegetarian diet. The health aspect of vegetarianism means a lot to me because I've also inherited the tendency toward high cholesterol and clogged arteries. I had my level taken before I was a vegetarian and it was 179, very high for a kid of 13. Now that I'm a strict vegetarian, it's down to 129.

There is not much you can do about the genes you inherited from your parents, but you do have a choice about what you will eat. Opting for vegetarianism is the best way to combat a family disposition toward high cholesterol, coronary artery disease, and cancer.

CANCER: According to the authors of *Becoming Vegetarian*, "One in four individuals in North America can expect to die of cancers. It is estimated that of these cancers, some 30–40 percent are diet-related in men, and as many as 60 percent are diet-related in women."[7] There are definite connections between what you eat and your chances of developing cancer, specifically the amount of fat. Vegetarians, as a group, tend to have much less fat in their diets and have a lower rate of cancer than nonvegetarians.

Points to keep in mind about cancer:

- ◇ People in affluent, "developed" nations like the United States and those of Western Europe eat the most meat and dairy products in the world, and, not coincidentally, have the highest rate of cancer in the world. People who live in "less developed" countries, like those in Asia and Africa, tend to have a much lower cancer rate.

- ◇ Studies done on vegetarians in Great Britain, Germany, Japan, and Sweden reveal that they have lower cancer mortality rates than meat eaters.

- ◇ Vegetarianism can help prevent several types of specific cancers, including breast, colon, liver, pancreas, uterus, prostate, and stomach cancer.

◇Many of the foods that a healthy vegetarian diet contains help prevent cancer. Among these "cancer-fighting" foods are the vegetarian staples: grains, vegetables, legumes, and fruits.

◇Some of the components in foods and the environment that are linked to different cancers are:

>   Fat (specifically trans-fatty acids and saturated acids)
>   Protein
>   Cholesterol
>   Pesticides
>   Food additives
>   Chemical changes in food preparation

◇Elements in the food you eat that can help prevent cancer include:

>   Fiber
>   Vitamins (A, C, D, E, folic acid)
>   Minerals (selenium, calcium, zinc, iron, copper)
>   Phytochemicals (certain chemicals found in plants)

We still do not know whether cancer is actually preventable. As with heart disease, there is a very strong genetic component involved with many types of cancer. However, study after study shows that a well-balanced vegetarian diet, one that includes ample fruits and vegetables, helps to forestall the disease.

HIGH BLOOD PRESSURE: High blood pressure is a condition that people generally develop as they get older. However, many young people have high blood pressure in countries where diets are rich in fat and cholesterol. It is not known exactly what component of the vegetarian diet keeps blood pressure at normal and low levels; however, scientists believe it is a combination of dietary factors (for example, eating a low-sodium diet), weight, and various plant substances.

DIABETES: There are two kinds of diabetes: type I and type II. Type I usually appears during childhood through early adulthood and requires daily doses of insulin, a life-supporting hormone or "chemical messenger." People who have type I diabetes no longer produce insulin, so they must inject it into their bodies to maintain their blood sugar levels. Type II diabetes generally appears in older people and can be controlled by taking pills and by modifying one's diet. Both forms of diabetes require people to maintain a healthy, low-fat diet and do plenty of exercise.

Health professionals increasingly recommend that people with diabetes adhere to a vegetarian diet to help prevent and treat the disease. A vegetarian plan is suggested because it is usually low in fat and high in both fiber and complex carbohydrates. There is still much research for scientists to do in this area, but so far they have found that:

- Low-fat, vegetarian diets help treat symptoms that result from diabetes, such as neuropathy (damage to nerves caused by high blood pressure).
- Lean, healthy people who eat diets very high in fat have been known to actually exhibit symptoms of mild diabetes. Even with limited research, scientists have discovered that vegetarians are less likely to show signs of diabetes than meat eaters.
- The protein in cow's milk may help trigger dia-

betes in children who are genetically predis-
posed to the disease.

Several factors are involved in the onset of diabetes, but a
diet that includes meat and dairy is certainly part of the
equation.

OSTEOPOROSIS: Osteoporosis is a disease in which bones
become less dense and more brittle over time due to calcium
loss. Scientists have found that osteoporosis is highly con-
centrated among women in Western Europe and the United
States. In the United States alone, somewhere between 15
and 20 million people have osteoporosis. As we have noted,
people in highly developed countries like the United States
also eat more fat and protein than anywhere else in the world.
This has led researchers to look at how diet may affect osteoporosis. What they have found is that a high intake of protein
can actually cause the body to *lose* calcium.

◇When you eat meat and other animal proteins,
you generally produce a dangerous acidic condition in your blood. Your body tries to neutral-
ize this acid in different ways. One of these is to
release calcium from the bones to wash the acid
out of your blood. Unfortunately, this also
washes out the calcium through the urine.

◇We are constantly told by the dairy industry that
milk is the best way to get calcium, which is
necessary for such bodily functions as muscle
contraction, nerve transmission, and blood clot-
ting. The truth is that you can get plenty of calcium from vegetables, grains, and legumes, and
bypass all the fat and hormones in most commercially sold dairy products.

Studies conducted on women in Asia, where people ingest no cow's milk and eat very little if any meat, show that there is almost no incidence of osteoporosis. They get plenty of calcium, but none of it from dairy products.

LACTOSE INTOLERANCE: Many people in the world, including those in Asia and Africa, are unable to digest cow's milk because they lack an enzyme called *lactase*. Every human is born with enough lactase to digest the sugar in its mother's milk (*lactose*), but the enzyme drops to an almost nonexistent level by age 5. If you cannot digest dairy products, then you are lactose intolerant. When lactose-intolerant people ingest milk, they can experience severe stomach pains, gas, and diarrhea.

More and more people are discovering that they cannot digest milk and that giving up dairy products actually makes them feel much healthier. Some people argue that drinking cows milk is foolish to begin with. If you compare the size of cows to that of humans, why would anyone think we need their milk (intended for their babies) to survive? With a little effort you can discover a great variety of foods that have all the nutrients found in milk and other dairy products.

OBESITY: Vegetarians, as a group, tend to be a lean bunch. They tend to stick to a low-fat, high-carbohydrate diet, one that is most efficient at preventing disease and promoting longevity. Obesity is a condition that currently affects about 20 million American children and is caused by a combination of factors. Obesity, scientists have discovered, is partly due to genetics, meaning it can run in families. However, people tend to be overweight because they eat too much fat and do not exercise enough.

Interestingly, some studies show that vegetarians eat as many calories as meat eaters and do not exercise as much.

Obviously it is not *how much* they eat, but *what* they eat that keeps vegetarians slim and healthy. If you exercise and cut excess fat from your diet—and becoming a vegetarian is a good way to achieve this—you will probably lose unwanted pounds.

HORMONES: Among other reasons, 18-year-old Jason Sanyas became a vegetarian because he "found out that beef, pork, and chicken have a lot of artificial hormones injected into them. I read a lot of health magazines and saw a news report on beef in the United States, and after that, I decided that's it, no more meat." Jason is absolutely correct: The meat and dairy industries in this country administer an excessive amount of hormones to livestock.

Naturally occurring hormones such as insulin and progesterone do amazing things in our bodies. Unfortunately, meat and dairy farmers use hormones to fatten animals unnaturally and extend their breeding cycles. These hormones go straight into the meat and dairy products that are sold in stores and restaurants. Many of these substances—such as DES (diethylstilbestrol), which is used to fatten and tenderize animals—are very harmful to humans and are known to cause cancer.

ANTIBIOTICS: Livestock animals, as we have read, live under very stressful conditions and often do not survive until they are slaughtered. In order to avoid constant sickness and infection, farmers administer enormous doses of antibiotics. In fact, Gary Null reports in his book, *The Vegetarian Handbook: Eating Right for Total Health:* "Since they were first introduced into animal feed in 1949, the use of antibiotics has grown from 490,000 pounds in 1954, to 1.2 million in 1960, to around 9 million pounds today."[8]

You and I take these medicines if we have strep throat or bronchitis, but not all the time. One of the problems with giving so many antibiotics to livestock is that the bacteria that cause the specific infection become immune to the specific antibiotic due to overexposure to the drug. Farmers then have to use even greater doses or different types of antibiotics to prevent illness.

Needless to say, when we eat animals treated with so many antibiotics or drink their milk, we ingest these substances as well. We can even become resistant to the antibiotics needed to treat such bacterial infections as *E. coli* and salmonella simply by eating infected meat.

ADDITIVES AND PESTICIDES: It can take quite some time for meat to arrive on your table after slaughter. In order to keep it from decaying too rapidly, the meat industry uses chemical additives. They also use dyes to make the meat look healthier, fresher, and redder than it would otherwise. Some of the most common additives are a group of preservatives known as sodium nitrites and sodium nitrates, which are found in most hot dogs and lunch meats. Several studies show that these toxic substances cause cancer. Sadly, they are not the only ones. The list includes:

◇Monosodium glutamate (a flavor enhancer)

◇BHT (used to prevent meat fat from becoming rancid)

◇BHA (also used to prevent rancidity)

◇Red Dye #2 (banned by the Food and Drug Administration)

The only way to be sure you are not eating any of these additives is to not eat any commercially prepared meat or animal products. If you are still eating some meat, organic and certain free-range meats are obviously a better, healthier choice, as they will at least be free of chemical additives.

Pesticides are another hidden health danger. Animals carry these toxic, cancer-causing substances around in their bodies after ingesting contaminated food. We in turn consume these chemicals when we eat a steak or a chicken leg from these animals. Nearly 100,000 Americans suffer the effects of pesticide poisoning each year, which can include exhaustion, headaches, fever, and muscle aches. There are hundreds of these dangerous pesticides, but the most familiar is DDT. By some estimates, "60 percent of cattle, 80 percent of poultry, and nearly 40 percent of swine are contaminated with the pesticide DDT, yet these animals are found to be fit legally for human consumption."[9]

Again, if you do not consume animal products, then you will not eat the pesticides stored in their meat and milk. However—and this is a real concern for vegetarians and meat eaters alike—many fruits, grains, and vegetables can contain the same dangerous pesticides as meat. One way for vegetarians to reduce this serious health risk is to wash vigorously (some recommend using soap!) everything you eat before you cook it. A better, healthier, but often more expensive or difficult-to-find alternative is to buy only those fruits, grains, and vegetables that are certified organic. Certified organic products have been grown using soil, water, sunlight, and natural fertilizers. As such, they are more or less guaranteed not to contain any harmful additives, hormones, or dangerous pesticides.

BETTER HEALTH FOR EVERYONE

Contrary to popular opinion, teens are interested in their health; they just need to know the facts. Danielle Pierce, 19, says:

I started thinking about becoming a vegetarian when I was in eighth grade. One of my teachers made a presentation about health and mentioned the healthy aspects of cutting down on meat. She really opened my eyes. It was the first time that I had ever actually heard or thought about meat as a health issue.

Remember, when you stop eating animal products, you are not only helping animals, but you are also taking a major step to improving your health now and into the future.

ENVIRONMENT

THE MANY VARIED reasons for becoming a vegetarian are all interconnected. Anyone who is interested in the state of the environment is certainly aware of this fact. People say they are vegetarians for ethical reasons without sometimes realizing that their choice affects the natural world as well. I have been to the Latin American country of Costa Rica several times and have seen the effects of rain forest destruction. Why does Costa Rica cut down so much of its natural treasure? To raise cattle for hamburgers.

UPSETTING THE NATURAL BALANCE

Few things disturb the natural order more than raising livestock. The waste in resources is enormous and the loss of land potentially irreversible. Some of the environmental costs that are ultimately due to a demand for animal products include:

DEFORESTATION: Much of the beef for the United States is raised in Central and South America and then shipped to the

United States. Countries such as Brazil, Argentina, and Costa Rica have some of the world's largest rain forests, which are home to the greatest biodiversity on the entire planet—literally millions of varied plant and animal species. The rain forests also provide us with oxygen, moderate the earth's climate, act as a defense against soil erosion, and prevent floods. Many of these nations are cutting down their precious rain forests to make grazing lands for cattle. Central American countries had 130,000 square miles of virgin rain forest in 1960, when the United States began importing beef from them. Now, less than 80,000 remain. Experts estimate that at this rate, in 40 years the rain forests will be entirely destroyed.

SOIL EROSION: When ranchers clear land for cattle grazing, it contributes to the erosion of soil, a process known as *desertification.* The dark top layer of soil is nutrient-rich, holds moisture, and is essential for plant growth. When the cattle feed on the land, they further contribute to the loss of soil by eating the plants that keep this layer of dirt firmly in place. When the soil is loose, the wind blows the layers off, making it impossible to hold water and grow more food for the animals. Replenishing the soil after it has eroded is not only difficult but expensive. Usually ranchers move on to other pieces of land rather than working with the one they have depleted.

WATER WASTE: Water is necessary for life. Many industries waste enormous amounts of water, but few so gratuitously as the meat and dairy industries. In the United States alone, over half of all the water consumed is used to irrigate land for animal feed and fodder. Amazingly, it takes 2,500 gallons of water to produce one pound of meat and 4,000 gallons to make one day's food for a meat eater. It takes only

300 gallons of water for a vegetarian's total daily requirement. Many people are unaware that there is a water crisis in several parts of the world. To waste so much of this precious resource raising animals we do not need to eat is truly shortsighted, not to mention selfish.

ECONOMICS

Less than half the harvested agricultural acreage in the United States is used to grow food for people.

—John Robbins

When you choose a vegetarian lifestyle, you are not only doing something positive for animals, your body, and the environment, but you are also helping to feed the rest of world. The meat and dairy industries are big businesses. In fact, one of the reasons that animals are treated in such a senseless and cruel fashion is that they are viewed by people in the industry only as money-making machines. Livestock farmers are interested in growing food for their animals, not for other people. Unfortunately, a lot of the land used for animal feed could be much better used to produce healthy grains, vegetables, fruits, and legumes for much of the world's hungry human population.

WHAT'S MONEY GOT TO DO WITH IT?

There are several areas where producing animal products and economics intersect. Here is a short list of some of them:

ANIMALS EAT A LOT: There are many places in the world where people are starving, including parts of Africa, India, and Asia. There are also areas all over the planet where people do not get enough to eat each day, including the United States, Central and South America, and Russia. Instead of using land to grow food for people, farmers use it either to graze animals or to produce livestock feed. Livestock in the United States consume "enough grain and soybeans to feed over five times the entire human population of the country."[10] Animals also consume over 80 percent of the corn and 95 percent of the oats we grow.

WASTED LAND: Farmers can much more efficiently use the land devoted to raising beef cattle and other food animals to grow food for people. Most of you probably think that the reason hunger exists in the world is because there is not enough food, but this is not true. Not enough land is allotted for people because the powerful meat and dairy industries want it for their money-making machines. The U.S. Department of Agriculture states that "one acre of land can grow 20,000 pounds of potatoes. That same acre of land, if used to grow cattlefeed, can produce less than 165 pounds of beef."[11] Essentially, land that is used to raise food for cattle provides less food than does land that is used to grow plants.

SO MUCH ENERGY: Making meat not only wastes land, water, soil, and food that people could eat, but it also takes a lot of costly energy to produce the final supermarket product. Before a steak makes its way to someone's dinner plate, farmers have shipped the animal by truck or train to a slaughterhouse, and then the meat is transported to a warehouse or store. All this moving around takes a lot of energy and costs a lot of money. One of the reasons meat is so expensive is because of the energy it takes to transport animals and meat. Author Frances Moore Lappé reports:

A detailed 1978 study sponsored by the Department of Interior and Commerce produced startling figures showing that the value of raw materials consumed to produce food from livestock is greater than the value of all oil, gas, and coal consumed in [the United States].[12]

As you can see, eating animal products is profitable for the people who own the meat and dairy companies, and they work toward making more money all the time. Unfortunately, while they prosper, a lot of the world's population goes to bed hungry every night.

RELIGION

And God said, Behold, I have given you every herb bearing seed, which is upon the face of all the earth, and every tree, in which is the fruit of a tree yielding seed; to you it shall be for meat.

—Genesis 1:29

ACCORDING TO THE Old Testament of the Bible, God decided that in the Garden of Eden, Adam and Eve would be vegetarians. There was no need to eat animals, as he had supplied them with so many other wonderful things to eat. It was not until Eve ate a forbidden apple and they were banished from Eden by God that they began to eat their fellow earthdwellers.

Many of the world's great religions either forbid or restrict the eating of meat and dairy products. Teens who grow up in homes where meat is not consumed for religious reasons have their first experience with vegetarianism within the family.

CHRISTIANITY

Different groups of Christians have their own sets of rules regarding diet (for example, some Catholics do not eat meat on Fridays), but there is not an official policy of vegetarianism. As discussed earlier, the Seventh-Day Adventists have long been strong proponents of vegetarianism in the United States. They want to eat the healthiest diet possible; and abstaining from meat is one way they can achieve this goal.

JUDAISM

Heather Mandel's family is Jewish and keeps a kosher home. This means that they have many rules about what they do and do not eat according to the Jewish teachings. Her family is not strictly vegetarian, but as she says, "there are limits to what we can eat. Coming from a kosher family definitely made the transition to vegetarianism much easier. I was already used to limiting what I put in my mouth." There are many historical reasons why the ancient Jews did not eat meat. Some believed that because flesh food was considered desirable, not to have it was a good punishment. Others saw eating meat as unclean and an act of gluttony. In addition, ancient cooking techniques were often unsanitary; certain flesh foods, like pork and shellfish, spread disease. This, along with numerous other reasons, led to the enactment of ancient kosher laws.

ISLAM

Some rituals in Islam require the slaughtering of animals. Historically, however, some adherents embraced vegetarianism because they believed it cruel to destroy defenseless animals. One sect of Islam, the Sufis, practices vegetarianism because it promotes their belief in a simple and austere life.

HINDUISM

According to sacred Hindu doctrines, "[m]eat can never be obtained without injury to living creatures."[13] This Indian religion believes that its adherents should abstain from eating flesh because it is cruel to animals and unhealthy to the spirit. Jason Sanyas, whose family comes from India, became a vegetarian partially for health reasons and partially for religious reasons. His family members are not strict vegetarians, but he says, "According to my Hindu origins, it's a sin to eat meat and for me that's important to remember."

BUDDHISM

Interestingly, while Buddhists believe that followers of the religion should not destroy living beings, kill, steal, or lie or practice a host of other sins, Buddhism is rather ambiguous about eating meat. Apparently the Buddha devised a rationale for eating meat: followers were not allowed to eat flesh that someone killed expressly for them, but they could eat meat that was already dead. Needless to say, complete abstinence from meat has long been a controversy in the Buddhist religion.

Many other religions have their own specific and idiosyncratic ideas about their followers' diets, but most do have some clause about abstaining from meat at some point during the year.

No Taste For Meat

SIXTEEN-YEAR-OLD JENNY ORVIS, who stopped eating meat when she was 3, says, "I just never liked the taste of meat." She says that everyone in her school knew she was a vegetarian and that they were very respectful about her decision. It is true that some kids are born without a desire to eat meat. They proceed through their early life ideally eating a healthier and more balanced diet than their peers, only to discover later that there are a wealth of other good reasons for not eating meat. As Jenny states, "I didn't really become a vegetarian because of the whole animal issue, but as I progressed I became more aware and involved."

Media Influence

TEENS ARE GREATLY influenced by the seemingly ever-present media frenzy around them. How can they not be when television, movies, books, magazines, rock concerts, sporting events, and the radio are such a big part of their life? Many teens become vegetarians because they feel it is cruel to mistreat and kill animals for food, but often they first begin to think about these issues after hearing a famous person talk about vegetarianism.

TELEVISION

If you've ever watched the popular television show *Roseanne,* you have no doubt heard Sara Gilbert's character speak out against the "meat-industrial complex." [14] Gilbert is just one of many celebrities who use their star power and influence to promote their views that eating meat is not cool.

She stated in *Tiger Beat* magazine, "I've been a vegetarian for three years for ethical, environmental, and health reasons. . . . I encourage other teenagers to inform themselves about animal issues because they are tied to the environment, our own health and our ethics."[15]

MOVIES

Babe, a movie about a young pig who performs some amazing feats, has done a lot to push many would-be vegetarians over the edge. Jill Edelman, 20, says, "I always toyed with the idea of becoming a vegetarian, but after seeing *Babe*, I was convinced." Other movies that portray animals in intelligent and sympathetic roles help change attitudes about what people eat.

MUSIC

Vegetarians also abound in the music scene. Gina Vivinetto wrote in the *St. Petersburg Times*, "At 14 I listened to so many songs by the Smiths that changed my life . . . because their songs crystallized for me the grim reality of slaughterhouses. When Morrissey said *Meat is Murder* it fostered sentiments in me that erupted in a holiday flip-out. . . . It was Easter and I asked my mom where the ham came from."[16] The Smiths' famous album did influence a number of teens, but do not forget that R.E.M.'s lead singer Michael Stipe and former 10,000 Maniacs lead singer Natalie Merchant are both fervent spokespeople for the cause, as is Pearl Jam's Eddie Vedder, veteran rocker David Bowie, and Madonna.

ATHLETES

Parents may not feel that these role models are the picture of health, but when teens inform Mom and Dad that athletes such as skater Surya Bonaly, wrestler Chris Campbell, and tennis player Martina Navratilova are also vegetarians, they may feel a little more reassured.

MAGAZINES

Many publications, including *Vegetarian Times* and *How on Earth*, publish articles, essays, and recipes that are very helpful when you are trying to start and maintain your vegetarian lifestyle. After reading about the death of actor River Phoenix (albeit from a drug overdose), teen Petra Bibeau decided to give up meat. She says, "It really impressed me that he felt we should respect animals as equals."[17]

BOOKS

A seminal work about the horrors of the meat industry is Upton Sinclair's *The Jungle*. It should be required reading for anyone interested in vegetarianism and animal rights. In fact the portrait Sinclair painted of the unsanitary, inhumane, and often downright revolting practices then prevalent in the meat industry prompted a series of laws and reforms in the 1920s.

On another level, who can forget the timeless story of Wilbur the pig in E. B. White's classic children's book *Charlotte's Web*? The book presented a humane picture of a farm animal that was smart, funny, and very lovable. Books can convey positive models, as well as a wealth of information, for kids and teens who want to be vegetarians.

There is no doubt that the media touch all of our lives every day. Ideally, what we see, hear, and read helps us to make positive decisions about how we choose to live. When celebrities, athletes, and writers help teens learn about the positive aspects of vegetarianism, they are using their star power in the best possible way.

PEER PRESSURE

NO ONE UNDERSTANDS peer pressure better than teenagers. If someone in a crowd wants to try something unusual, he or she is often shunned because it is generally not cool to be different. As Elana Adams says, "It's hard to be a vegetarian when everyone around you makes you feel bad because you're not eating meat." People want approval from their peers, especially during adolescence. Many vegetarian teens, while strong in their convictions, still want respect from their friends and classmates. Increasingly, vegetarianism is now considered an acceptable (even *cool*!) option for image-conscious teens. As 14-year-old Allison Reid-Cunningham says, "There's a big new trend, a big wave of teen-age vegetarians. . . . It's more . . . acceptable."[18]

Vegetarianism is growing so popular that some teens are concerned that the whole vegetarian movement might just be getting *too* trendy. Joanna Helmuth, 15, of St. Louis, Missouri, fears that vegetarianism "is becoming a big thing to do—save the world, become a vegetarian. I'm a vegetarian because I don't like meat, not because I want to be popular."[19] Chances are, if you choose vegetarianism only because it is something all your friends are doing, you will not stay a vegetarian for long. Being a vegetarian takes sacrifice, awareness, and hard work. It is not something to do casually for any reason.

TEENAGE REBELLION

WHEN YOU ANNOUNCE to your parents that you are becoming a vegetarian, they may roll their eyes, put their hands over their mouths, or shake their heads in disbelief. Chalking it all up to some adolescent phase, they may not understand, or want to admit, that by doing something different from them, you are beginning to assert your independence.

You may also decide that a little teenage rebellion is not such a bad thing and stop eating meat just to show them you have some control over your life. Mike Ravitz explains, "I think teens like [vegetarianism] because it is radical and has elements of rebellion. It's not just a fad, but for many it really goes right to their soul, right to who they are." To put it another way, Jessica Almy, 17, states, "What we eat is one thing we can have control over."[20]

Petra Bibeau did not become a vegetarian to make her parents angry, but she certainly exhibited a rebellious streak each time the family would sit down to dinner. Her mother states, "We'd be eating meat and she'd sit there and make grotesque faces, saying 'That was a living thing—it could be grazing in a pasture.'" Her sister, Claudine Bibeau, states, "It would ruin our appetites and gross us out."[21]

Petra and her family were eventually able to find a middle ground, but many teens continue to battle with their parents over diet in their pursuit of some degree of independence. We will look at how teen vegetarians and their families can co-exist in Chapter 4.

VEGETARIAN PARENTS

SOME TEENS ARE vegetarians because their parents do not eat or cook meat. In the 1960s many people sought an alternative lifestyle that included omitting animal products from their diets, a practice they, in turn, passed on to their children. Health guru Gary Null states, "Role models . . . are imperative if a child is to be given a choice,"[22] and parents need to be these models.

Parents may promote a vegetarian diet at home, but that does not mean their children will follow it forever. *The Vegetarian Alternative* author Vic Sussman states that one mother asked him, "'But how can I make sure my children will stay vegetarians?' He replies, "You can't, no more than you can insure their absolute adherence to your religious beliefs or moral values."[23] Generally, however, when parents provide a healthy example, their children grow up and mimic this model.

If your parents are vegetarians and you feel they are pushing you into being one yourself, beware. Take a step back and try to figure out whether this is something you want to do or something you are doing because your parents are pressuring you to do so. Sussman warns, "[I]t's so important to keep vegetarianism in perspective. Parents who push too hard—teaching their children that meat eaters are gross or bloodthirsty—may end up raising herbivorous bigots who *invite* anger and ridicule."[24] People change their habits, especially their eating habits, through education and awareness, not through coercion.

EATING DISORDERS

THERE IS ONE dangerous reason why teens choose to stop eating meat: They want to stop eating food altogether. The adolescent years are full of all kinds of pressure and one of those, especially for teenage girls, is to be thin. One way they try to achieve this goal is to become a vegetarian because meat is just one more thing they can eliminate from their daily diet.

Anorexia is an eating disorder in which a person, usually a young woman, stops eating food because she thinks she is too fat. According to an article in *Newsweek*, "[M]any young women who suffer from anorexia start out as vegetarians. . . . For anorectics, giving up meat is an inconspicuous, socially acceptable way to cut down on calories"[25] Pre-med student Bonnie Sherman gave up meat when she was 15 and by 17 ate only carrots. She lost 40 pounds and still eats mainly bagels and frozen yogurt.[26] Psychologist Perry Belfer, director of the Newton-Wellesley Hospital eating disorder center in Massachusetts, notes that people who begin a restrictive diet, such as vegetarianism, can be on their way to an eating disorder.

Nutritionist and dietitian Brenda Davis estimates that 50 percent of teenage vegetarians are anorexic. She explains:

The way to tell whether a person is really veggie or suffering from an eating disorder, is their willingness to consume vegetarian foods that are higher in fat and calories and if they are willing to eat beans, nuts, tofu, and seeds. Most anorexics would not touch a nut. If they are refusing all these things, it's really a red light and you have to question their motives. If you're choosing it for health you should be willing to balance it a bit. So many anorexics are vegetarians because it legitimizes what they're doing.

If you suspect that someone you know has anorexia, speak to either your parents or a school health official about what to do. Anorexia does not generally just go away. It can lead to severe, long-lasting health problems or even death, and people who have it need therapy and counseling to figure out why they are not eating.

YOU HAVE MADE YOUR DECISION

YOU HAVE RESEARCHED the reasons, stated your case, and now friends and family know: You are going to be a vegetarian. Your next step, and perhaps their next question, is to find out what type of vegetarian you want to be. Most experts agree that whatever you choose, taking it slowly is the best way to make the transition. In Chapter 3, we will look at the different kinds of vegetarians.

— 3 —

IS THERE ONLY ONE KIND OF VEGETARIAN?

There never were in the world two opinions alike, no more than two hairs or two grains; the most universal quality is diversity.

—Montaigne, sixteenth-century
French philosopher

THE term *vegetarian* means something different for everyone. Just as no two people are the same, there is not one "correct" way to be a vegetarian. When teens decide they want to try removing certain items from their diets, perhaps starting with meat or dairy products, people often ask: What kind of vegetarian do you want to be? Hopefully your first answer will be, "A healthy one."

THE THREE BASICS

THERE ARE THREE basic types of vegetarians that you may have heard about. They are:

◇Lacto-ovo

◇Lacto

◇Vegan

In addition to these commonly used terms, you may come across people who refer to themselves as:

◇Semivegetarians

◇Macrobiotics

◇Omnivores

These are general terms that doctors, nutritionists, and writers use to classify groups of people into dietary categories, but they may not be the only ones you come across. You might meet a person who calls himself a pesco vegetarian or a fruitarian. We will discuss these and other terms later in this chapter.

So remember: It is somewhat important to know what type of vegetarian diet you want to follow, if for no other reason than to tell people when they ask you! Get all the information you can on each type and then make your decision based on your research. The best overall approach is to not rush into a diet where you feel that you are depriving yourself of something delicious. If you feel something missing in your diet or are tempted by the food you have stopped eating, then you probably are not ready to truly let go. You want to enjoy your food, not resent the fact that you do not eat hamburgers. Keep in mind what artist Sue Coe emphasizes: that you should be "doing the best you can."

KEEPING THE EGGS AND DAIRY: THE LACTO-OVO DIET

MOST TEENS START out as lacto-ovo vegetarians, which means they continue to eat eggs and dairy products, for three simple reasons:

⬦They have more foods to choose from.

⬦Even if they intend to lead a strict vegetarian lifestyle later on, giving up so many foods at once can be difficult.

⬦Most people do not know enough about a strict vegan diet.

In most cases, new vegetarian teenagers are advised to keep eating eggs and dairy products to ensure that they will still get enough fat, cholesterol, and calories on a regular basis. Of course, even if you are continuing to eat eggs and dairy products, be advised that too much can definitely be a bad thing.

VARIETY

"Giving up meat was not so hard," says 18-year-old Melissa Smith, "but not eating eggs and dairy is kind of tough." Eggs and dairy are very common and delicious ingredients in many foods, so giving them up is not always that easy. Manufacturers and chefs often use these items in cakes, breads, pancake mixes, and cookies. You can also prepare eggs in a variety of ways, including scrambling, boiling, and frying. Dairy products such as cheese, yogurt, ice cream, and butter are favorites during snacks and mealtimes. It is becoming much easier to find dairy products and eggs that come from animals raised on small, humane farms, and that are produced organically. Health food stores and even large supermarket chains offer hormone-free, pesticide-free, and antibiotic-free milk, cheese, yogurt, and ice cream, as well as organic eggs.

HEALTH

Lacto-ovo vegetarians avoid eating all meat, poultry, and fish, which are traditional sources for much of the protein we eat. However, eggs and dairy products are sources of complete protein, containing sufficient amounts of the essential amino acids we need to eat. But be aware that certain dairy products, like butter and milk, are poor sources of protein and contain enormous amounts of fat. Your best sources of protein as a lacto-ovo vegetarian are eggs and cheese. Eggs and most dairy products also contain vitamin B-12, which is essential for nerve function and cell division. We will talk more about why B-12 is an issue for strict vegetarians and vegans in a later chapter.

THINK SKIM

If you are going to eat dairy products, one way to ensure that you get the nutritional value without all of the fat is to eat a certain portion of low-fat or no-fat dairy products. Of course, as you will find out later, many plant sources can provide much of the nutrition obtained from both dairy and eggs without the attendant health risks.

HOLD THE EGGS: THE LACTO DIET

LACTO VEGETARIANS NOT only stop eating meat, chicken, and fish, but they also eliminate eggs from their diets. This is a bit more challenging than the lacto-ovo diet because so many products, such as cakes and cookies, contain eggs in their ingredients. "I thought when I was going to give up eggs," says Elana Adams, "that it would be easy. I don't really like eggs for breakfast or at any other time. What I didn't think about was all the other foods that *contain* eggs."

HEALTH

Eggs are a good source of protein, much better than any dairy product, but the yellow yolk is very high in cholesterol. As a result, when you stop eating them, you will eliminate a lot of cholesterol from your diet. As an added ethical benefit, you are also protesting against the egg-laying practices described in Chapter 2. As with the lacto-ovo diet, you do not have to worry about B-12 because dairy products contain this life-sustaining vitamin.

DAILY DAIRY NEEDS

Eliminating eggs is a great step toward total vegetarianism, if that is where you are headed, but do not then binge on all the cheese, ice cream, and yogurt you can get your hands on. While dairy products do contain some essential nutrients, their presence in our diets has been, as Dudley Giehl says in *Vegetarianism: A Way of Life,* "grossly exaggerated by the dairy industry."[1]

HOLD EVERYTHING: THE VEGAN DIET

MANY VEGETARIAN TEENS are "going all the way"; that is to say, they are completely eliminating all animal products not only from their diets, but also from their wardrobes and cosmetic cases. Some refer to veganism as "strict vegetarianism" or "total vegetarianism," but these terms seem very limiting to me. If you are a vegan, even with its stringent rules of "dos and don'ts," you can still create your own definition. The following is a partial list of products that some vegans do not use:

◇Honey
◇Leather
◇Fur
◇Wool
◇Feathers
◇Perfume

◇ Animal-tested cosmetics

◇ Animal-tested household products

Of course, vegans also do not eat meat, chicken, fish, dairy products, or eggs.

What's Hiding in My Food?

If you want to embrace veganism from the start, although it is advisable to start slowly, keep in mind all the places you will have to look for animal products. Watch for:

◇ Commercially baked goods, including bread, cookies, cakes, and muffins, which often contain eggs and dairy products.

◇ Cheese can contain a substance called rennet, from the lining of a cow's stomach. Make sure that the cheese you buy is suitable for vegans— such as soy cheese.

◇ Vegetarian burgers may use eggs for binding.

◇ Soy cheese manufacturers sometimes add a milk protein to make their cheese easier to melt.

It may take time, but as you begin to become a savvier shopper, you will more than likely be able to spot the hidden elements in food that you do not want to eat. If you are in a well-stocked health food store, but are a little confused, ask a clerk or manager to help you and always remember to read labels. Food manufacturers are required to list all the ingredients contained in their products. Fewer and fewer are using animal fats in their baked goods, but it is always important to check.

THE BEST FOR HEALTH

There is no question that for health and ethical reasons, the vegan diet is the best choice. It is a diet generally low in fat, cholesterol, and unnecessary protein, but one that also contains lots of fiber, grains, vegetables, fruits, nuts, and legumes. We are conditioned through traditional diet patterns to seek most of our zinc, vitamin D, protein, and calcium from animal sources. With a little effort, however, you can get all of these from plant sources. You will probably have to search and explore a bit more, but as Virginia and Mark Messina say in their book, *The Vegetarian Way*, "that's half the fun of a vegan diet."[2]

ONE TEEN'S SAGA

Gina Vivinetto writes in "I Was a Teenage Vegan" of some feelings and issues surrounding the delicate issue of teens and veganism:

The more I learned, the more I cringed until I questioned the whole issue: "Mother's milk is from a mom. My mom is a lady, not a cow." I am not now nor have I ever been a baby cow. Adult cows don't drink cow milk, why should I? The whole thing seemed crazy. Eggs and dairy products were phased out of my diet. So were any products with even traces of the stuff in it.

That meant no more cheese (sigh), no more ice cream, no more supermarket cookies (Have you ever read the ingredients in a bag of Oreos? They have lard and dairy products in them). Yogurt was out as was all my mom's homemade lasagna and pizza and her huge platters of mac 'n' cheese. What was cool was that this meant no more *Fat Me*. Although dairy products contain important vitamins and nutrients, many are also high in fat and cholesterol.

I was now a full-fledged vegan, give or take an occasional teaspoon of honey. A true vegan (pronounced VEE-gun) partakes of no products derived from any animal source. My closets were rid of leather and fur. My conscience felt a lot better. . . . I was spending my allowance on tofu.[3]

Gina was obviously willing to sacrifice a lot, and she went through hard times with both family and friends. She made her decision based on intense research and heightened awareness of both the health and ethical considerations involved in veganism. If you are going to try being a vegan, hers is a fine model to follow.

A GOOD WAY TO START: SEMIVEGETARIANISM

SOME TEENS ARE not ready to give up all of the animal products in their lives. Often, they are not even ready to give up most of them. That is okay because many people move into vegetarianism gradually, and becoming a semivegetarian is a positive step. As writer Debbie Salomon puts it, "Semivegetarians make substitutions based on common sense and good taste, not nutritional harangue."[4]

There are no set rules for semivegetarians; just about anything goes. Your goal is to start moderating certain foods in your diet. Start to limit how many hamburgers, hot dogs, and chicken wings you eat each week, and gradually cut meat out of your diet without feeling deprived. Most people begin by giving up red meat (steak, hamburger, lamb chops) and pork (bacon, sausage, pork chops), but continue to eat chicken and fish. But do what feels right for you. Again, each individual choosing vegetarianism does it in his or her own way. Deciding to go vegetarian is a choice you're making for yourself; how you get there is a personal choice too.

Another way to ease into vegetarianism is to try one new food a week. Let's say you have never tried baked ziti or lasagna without chopped meat. Find a recipe or ask someone in your family or a neighbor who knows how to cook and begin finding out the ingredients. Start with simple foods, like spaghetti and sauce with a big salad for dinner or brown rice and black beans with a sliced-tomato salad. You will probably find that you and your family are eating an altogether healthier diet.

If you go too fast, you may start missing meat and want to return to eating roast chicken, lamb, and bacon. That's okay too. Fifteen-year-old Meredith Visco gave up meat for two months before she started again. "Some foods I couldn't give up—like steak."[5] She now eats a moderate amount of meat and her family has cut back from eating meat five times a week to two.

A DIETARY PHILOSOPHY: MACROBIOTICS

AS WITH MOST forms of vegetarianism, the macrobiotic philosophy strives to create a sustainable and healthy system of eating for both people and the environment. Macrobiotics tend to consume locally grown foods to support local farmers and small agricultural ventures. Food is harvested and eaten according to its growing season, so in summer many fresh vegetables and fruits are plentiful, while in the fall and winter, grains and squashes are more readily available and easily preserved.

WHAT TO EAT?

Whole grains are the focus of meals, which can make up 50 to 60 percent of the macrobiotic diet. Vegetables fill in another 25 percent or so. If you adhere to this plan, the rest of what you eat consists of beans and small amounts of fruit, nuts, seeds, and occasionally some seafood and even meat or chicken. Other restrictions include vegetables from the nightshade family, which include potatoes, eggplant, and peppers. Macrobiotic eaters also abstain from tropical fruits and artificial sweeteners. They do not eat nightshade vegetables because most are not indigenous to the Americas and the plants are often used for such medicines as stimulants, narcotics, and pain relievers. They do not indulge in tropical fruits because of the high sugar content and growth in a foreign region. Artificial sweeteners are avoided because they are chemically produced and have no nutritional value.

HEALTH CONCERNS

While the macrobiotic diet has a number of health benefits, such as low-fat, mineral-rich foods and a lack of fatty or processed foods, it can be a nutritionally dangerous diet for growing children. Teens and children tend to need more fat and calories than this diet can provide. I would recommend that most teens do not try a macrobiotic diet unless they have very carefully researched their nutritional requirements and discussed them with a nutritionist.

EVERYTHING UNDER THE SUN: OMNIVORES

ANIMALS AND HUMANS are classified by what they eat, as you have read in this chapter. There is a term for probably every type of eating pattern and behavior that you can imagine. Some of the commonly known terms include:

◇ Carnivores—eat meat

◇ Herbivores—eat plants

◇ Omnivores—eat animal products and plants

There is considerable debate about whether humans are carnivores or herbivores by nature and design. Some scientists argue that due to the shape of our teeth, the length of our small intestine and colon, the type of our nails, and the kind of digestive enzymes in our saliva that we are simply not designed to eat meat. While the issue is hardly settled, there is little doubt that most people are omnivores by choice. If you are an omnivore, you eat meat, pork, chicken, fish, eggs, dairy products, vegetables, fruits, seeds, nuts, grains, legumes, and anything else you can safely ingest.

Obviously omnivores are not vegetarians, but in order to have a greater understanding of the issue as a whole and the spectrum of choices available, it is important to know about the many places where people can stand under the dietary umbrella.

OTHER TYPES OF VEGETARIANISM

YOU ARE NOW aware of several types of vegetarians and perhaps you have found a group that meshes with your dietary and ethical ideas. In addition to the types discussed earlier, there are several less commonly chosen subgroups that people have created to describe what they eat. They include:

◇ Ovo vegetarians

◇ Pesco vegetarians

◇ Pollo vegetarians

◆Hygienic vegetarians

◆Fruitarians (*not recommended*)

◆Sproutarians (*not recommended*)

◆Vitarians (*not recommended*)

◆Breathatarians (*not recommended*)

You are not limited by these terms and may discover a new category (for example, pesco-ovo vegetarian) that fits your own brand of vegetarianism. Remember that it is not the label you choose, but how responsibly you plan your diet that counts.

OVO VEGETARIANS

As you can probably guess, ovo vegetarians eat eggs, but not dairy products. In some ways this can potentially be a healthier choice than the lacto diet, because generally people eat fewer eggs than they do dairy products. A lacto vegetarian might have a bagel with cream cheese and a low-fat glass of milk for breakfast, a slice of pizza or a cheese sandwich for lunch, and for dinner a baked potato with butter, topped off by frozen yogurt for dessert. This is a lot of dairy for one day.

However, an ovo vegetarian might have an egg for breakfast, a few cookies and some bread that had eggs as part of their ingredients, perhaps a boiled egg for lunch on Wednesday, and maybe an omelet for dinner one night. It's harder to overdo it with eggs; it's unlikely that an ovo vegetarian could eat a quantity of eggs equal to the amount of dairy products that a lacto vegetarian could eat in one day.

HEALTH: Eggs have both health advantages and disadvantages. They are a complete protein food, meaning that they have all the essential amino acids that you need each day. The protein in eggs, contained in the white part, is far superior to any found in dairy products. Unfortunately, the yolk of an egg is the single highest source of dietary cholesterol.

FALSE ADVERTISING: Because eggs have so much cholesterol, they are not terribly heart-healthy. The fact that eggs and heart disease have been inextricably linked does not make egg producers very happy. To combat the image of the egg as an unhealthy choice, a group called the National Commission on Egg Nutrition published several booklets and ads claiming that risks of heart disease associated with eggs were untrue. The American Heart Association and several other health organizations filed a suit against the egg commission and their false practices. A judge ruled against the industry and denounced them for their deceptive practices.

It is always a good idea when you receive a pamphlet or booklet, whether about nutrition or something else, to find out who published the information. If you read a booklet distributed by the dairy industry professing that their cows lead a good life in the factory system, you have good reason to be skeptical.

In the end, however, if you choose to be an ovo vegetarian, then you need not worry about getting enough protein; even if you eat all of the egg, you will probably still eat much less fat and cholesterol overall than someone who eats meat and/or dairy products.

PESCO VEGETARIANS

A common form of vegetarianism for teens easing their way into a new diet is pesco vegetarianism, which means the only animal flesh you eat is fish. There are several reasons why this type is beneficial to both you and many of the animals that suffer in the factory system.

Chances are, unless there are anglers in your family, you do not eat fish every day. People generally eat much less seafood than they do other types of meat because fresh fish is often difficult to buy and often very expensive. A lot of families view fish as a food only for special occasions or for when company comes over. If you become a pesco vegetarian, yes, you will still be eating some type of animal, but probably far less than if you still ate beef, pork, or chicken.

One can also argue that fish that swim in oceans and rivers have a better quality of life until they are caught than do land animals in factories. For this reason, some pesco vegetarians feel that ethically it is better to eat fish caught in the ocean than other kinds of meat.

POLLO VEGETARIANS

Pollo vegetarians eat chicken, but no beef, pork, or fish. Most choose this option because chicken is easy to find, not terribly expensive, and easy to cook several different ways.

Chicken is a leaner meat than beef or pork, which makes it a healthier choice in terms of fat, but like all animal flesh it still contains saturated fat. It has an advantage over seafood in that it is less expensive and does not emit the strong odors that many kinds of fish do.

There are a few brands of "free-range" chickens on the market today, the most popular being Bell and Evans. Free-range chickens are not kept in cages, but allowed to roam in barnyards, ideally living according to their natural cycles until the time they are killed. Manufacturers of these birds do not use hormones or antibiotics, and they are for the most part free of chemical substances. They are a little more expensive and you may have to ask for them at a butcher shop, but short of certified-organic chickens, free-range is the best alternative.

HYGIENIC VEGETARIANS

Hygienic vegetarians don't eat meat but believe that animal by-products are all right to use. Essentially, if the animal is already dead, then it is deemed acceptable to use the remains. For example, a hygienic vegetarian will use a leather jacket made from a cow's hide, a goose-down comforter or jacket, or a feather pillow. You can be a lacto-ovo vegetarian, for example, and fall under this category, whereas another lacto-ovo may not agree with you on this subject.

In contrast, some vegetarians have no trouble eating eggs and dairy products, but will not use any products made using parts or materials from dead animals. They believe that even if you are only utilizing a by-product, you are encouraging the killing of animals for these items as well as for their meat.

The following vegetarian diets are splinter sects even within the subgroups listed here and are not recommended for teens or anyone else because of their lack of nutritional value.

FRUITARIANS

People choose to become fruitarians for various reasons and beliefs. Some think that it is a good way to lose weight fast because you're not eating very many calories. Unfortunately, you are also not getting enough nutrients either. Some prefer the taste of fruit, which is often very high in sugar, to that of other foods and feel less full after eating it.

Ethical fruitarians, who are concerned about what they call "plant consciousness," will not eat certain vegetables because the harvest destroys the entire plant. These include such foods as carrots, beets, turnips, and other tubers. However, they will eat fruits like tomatoes, legumes, apples, and melons, whose harvests do not involve killing the entire plant.

This diet is not recommended for teens or anyone else because there is no way to get all the nutrients you need in a day from eating fruit alone.

SPROUTARIANS

These vegetarians do not last very long on their meager diet of sprouted alfalfa, wheat, beans, and a few types of seeds. Sprouts, while nutritious along with a properly balanced meal, do not make a healthy diet by themselves.

VITARIANS

Another fringe group of vegetarians, vitarians will eat fruits and vegetables but will not eat seeds, nuts, or grains because they feel that these foods are unfit for human consumption. They proclaim their ideas based on philosophic and religious grounds.

BREATHATARIANS

This group, as its name suggests, purports that air is all people need to survive, and that food is unnecessary. The few adherents to this group make good newspaper stories, but also confirm many a parent's worst fears about extreme vegetarianism.

MAKING THE RIGHT CHOICE

YOU HAVE NOW read many of the options and I hope you are giving much thought to what type of vegetarian you want to be. As I have reiterated several times, it is best to start slowly when changing dietary habits, especially during adolescence, when you are growing so fast. Starting slowly also makes it easier for you to explore and experiment with new foods and cooking possibilities. Use the headings and information as guides, but feel free to become whatever kind of vegetarian you want. Ask as many questions as you need to and read as much literature as you can. There is no such thing as an overinformed vegetarian.

Ideally, you now know that you want to give vegetarianism a try and you have some good ideas about what types of food you may want to omit from your diet. In the next chapter we tackle the question of how you can be a vegetarian in a predominantly meat-eating society and lead a reasonably normal family and social life.

PART THREE

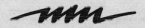

WHAT YOU NEED:
How to Lead a Happy and Healthy Vegetarian Life

4

How to Be a Vegetarian and Lead a Normal Life

Allow children to have freedom to make choices.

—Lena Romanoff, mother of a vegetarian

IF you decide that you want to pursue vegetarianism, then your life is going to change. Eating is generally a social time, one you spend with family or friends, talking about school or who scored the winning run during last night's big game. People have shared their meals for as long as they have been eating, and you are no different. So what happens when you suddenly stop choosing the foods that everyone else does? What happens when the questions start and all you want to do is concentrate on your beans and rice or salad? When you become a vegetarian, people are often suddenly very curious about your new diet.

One of the best ways to deal with the onslaught of questions and reactions to your vegetarianism is to be prepared. Read books, subscribe to magazines, go to workshops, and ask other vegetarian teens and adults how they managed when they switched over. Your family and friends may have any number of reasons for feeling that your vegetarianism is going to change your relationship with them. When you answer their concerns and queries with educated and non-threatening answers, generally life continues along without much hassle. You never know, they may even try it for themselves.

Some of the topics we will discuss in this chapter include:

◇ Parents
◇ Siblings
◇ Peers
◇ What to do when eating out
◇ How to manage the school cafeteria
◇ What to eat at other people's houses
◇ How to get through the holidays
◇ How to work around religious ceremonies
◇ When you are traveling
◇ If you are on a date
◇ When you are at camp
◇ Sports and vegetarianism
◇ Why support is so important
◇ Vegetarian diplomacy

PARENTS

CHANCES ARE, IF you are a teenager, you and your parents have had the occasional spat over what you wear, the length of your hair, what time you get home on a Saturday night, and what you eat. At one point or another, your parents have probably been concerned that you eat too much junk and not enough nutritious food. You can imagine their shock when you announce that you are now giving up, depending on what you decide, anything from just beef to all red meat, pork, chicken, fish, eggs, and dairy products.

ANNOUNCING YOU ARE A VEGETARIAN

Not all parents are the same, but most respond with some concern to their child's proposed dietary changes. When Lisa Ravitz's son Mike announced that he was going to be a vegetarian, she thought, "Fine, you give up meat, no big deal." But when Mike started to delve further into veganism, she occasionally got a little short-tempered with him. "I think our first argument was over honey," she says. "Honey to me seemed like a natural product, but then he told me that in most cases they kill the bees after the honey is produced and he would be no part of that."

Mike admits that sometimes it has been hard, but that overall, his parents have been very supportive of his decision. One thing that helped was that Mike learned as much as he could about vegetarianism before making his final choice and he gradually became a vegan over time. His mother now feels that "if a child is willing to sacrifice all they have to for a vegetarian lifestyle, then a parent should be willing to help them."

IT'S NOT JUST A PHASE

When you announce your big vegetarian news, your parents may roll their eyes and think, "Oh boy, here comes another phase." Remind them that changing your diet is not something you take lightly and that it is not just another passing fad. Sixteen-year-old Jenny Orvis says, "My parents thought it was a phase at first, something I was doing because it was trendy." Heather Mandel's parents also thought their daughter was just taking part in a typical teenage trend. She comments, "My parents found it a little annoying at times when I first started. My mom thought it was just a phase. Ironically, now we're kind of a veggie family. My mom makes me special food and then the rest of my family will eat it." The more facts you present to your parents, the easier it will be for them to realize that you are serious and educated about your choice.

NUTRITIONAL FEARS

The number one fear of most parents is that their child will not get adequate nutrition as a vegetarian. According to nutritionist Brenda Davis, "Parents are often quite concerned because they see their kids eating something like potatoes and corn, but not replacing the foods they've taken out, like meat and dairy." If you eliminate beef, chicken, and fish from your diet, you must replace the nutrients from these foods with foods like tofu, eggs, dairy products, and vegetables. Danielle Pierce, 19, relates:

> My mom was mostly concerned that I wouldn't get enough nutrients if I stopped eating meat. My doctor told me all the things that I could eat in place of meat. At a vegetarian camp I found all these recipes and simple dishes that I could make at home with my mom. I didn't get sick much after I became a vegetarian and stayed very active and my mom just got used to it. My dad had a hard time with it at first, but now he has also adjusted.

Tell your parents that you will consult with the family doctor or your pediatrician and a nutritionist if necessary. Make a list of all the foods that you will eat that have similar nutritional values as the ones you are omitting.

Nutritionist Maryanne Richardson suggests keeping a food diary to show your parents and your doctor that in fact you are eating five servings of fruit and vegetables each day, a reliable source of protein, enough carbohydrates, and a calcium-rich food. When you look back at your diary each week, you can see where you need to make adjustments for even healthier eating.

SO MANY MEALS TO PREPARE

Besides rolling their eyes, your parents may also let out a big groan and say, "How many meals are we going to have to cook for this family?" Preparing multiple dishes is one of the most commonly heard complaints from parents. Mike Ravitz says:

> Sometimes it's been hard because when my mom cooks dinner, she has to prepare three or four different meals because I'm a strict vegetarian, my dad and mom are different types of vegetarians, and so is my brother.

His mother, Lisa, concurs: "There are times when I find myself making four meals and if you're busy and harried, there's a bit of resentment."

Elizabeth Adams, Claire and Elana's mother, says, "Each meal consists of special dishes for the girls and then food for me and my husband. It would be easier if the girls helped out." Lending a hand in the kitchen, making your own meals, and even cooking dinner for the entire family one night a week are good ways to lift the more-than-one-meal-at-a-time burden off your parents' shoulders. Ways to help can include shopping with a parent at the supermarket or health food store, finding out which brands are least expensive and most nutritious, and looking through vegetarian cookbooks to find new and easy-to-prepare recipes.

Your parents may know very little about vegetarianism

and even less about vegetarian cooking. It will be up to you to educate them about how vegetarianism benefits not only your health, but also that of the entire family's.

CHALLENGING VALUES

Some parents can feel threatened by vegetarianism because they see it as a threat, both to their authority and to their ability to show love through food. Parents can have a very hard time when kids begin showing some independence and expressing their own values. Brenda Davis advises,

> With parents, the most important thing for children to do is to continue to respect their parents' values and not be critical of their choices. If you want your parents to respect your choices, you must respect theirs. Some parents may also feel a little threatened because so many traditions revolve around food.

Your parents have their own ideas about what they and you should eat, so perhaps a little compromise is not such a bad thing. Melissa Smith relates, "I was going to be a full vegetarian from the start, but my mother felt I needed some mainstay of protein, one that was easy to prepare. I'd not exactly been eating all the best protein substitutes in the beginning, so I agreed to eat fish."

Claire Adams talks about how she and her sister clashed with their parents in the beginning: "They gave us such a hard time when we started, it was very difficult. I think they were personally offended. They said, 'All right, don't eat meat, but you have to eat a lot of everything else.' They thought if we didn't eat five things at every meal, we would die. Now, several years later, they totally respect our decision." Generally, if you can avoid fighting with your parents about what you eat, then you will find it much easier not only to become a vegetarian, but also to stay one.

SUPPORTIVE PARENTS

You may be lucky and find that your parents are supportive of your decision from the moment you announce your new dietary status. Melissa Smith states, "My parents were supportive from the start. I became a vegetarian to lose weight and they thought it was a great idea, they just wanted me to be careful." Just as no two teenagers are alike, no two sets of parents will think or react the same way. If your parents support your vegetarianism, then show them that you truly know how to be a responsible and healthy one by taking as big a role in your nutrition as you can. It does take extra effort, but hopefully you realized when you decided to become a vegetarian that there would be a little more work involved around mealtime.

OPEN LINES OF COMMUNICATION

If your parents are concerned about your vegetarianism, remind them that you are taking responsibility for your actions. Suggest a few books for them to read, cook them a vegetarian feast, or show them the list of vegetarians past and present. Communication is central to your parents' understanding your commitment. If they still do not agree with you and want further confirmation that you are not making a foolish choice, have them call one of the many vegetarian support groups or a certified nutritionist.

Ideally, you will have shown your parents that you are well on your way to making well-planned and wise choices for yourself and the planet.

SIBLINGS

MANY PEOPLE ARE swayed by a vegetarian brother or sister. "I've been a vegetarian for a long time," says Jenny Orvis, "but my sister became one a few years ago. It's actually a lot easier for my parents now that both of us are vegetarians, because now we cook our own food." When more than one person in the house is a vegetarian, they can help each other prepare meals, shop, and figure out new foods to eat. Sisters Elana and Claire Adams became vegetarians at almost the same time and have helped each other deal with their parents' objections as well as peer pressure. "Sometimes," says Claire, "people used to tease us by putting hamburgers in our faces and saying, 'Look at the dumb cow.' It was really terrific to have my sister there for support."

Mike Ravitz, a vegan, is very proud of the fact that his parents are raising his baby brother as a vegetarian. He believes his brother began taking after him "when he first came home from the hospital and he had a problem digesting the baby formula, which was cow's milk. We switched him to soy formula and he's fine. I like to think he's already emulating his big brother."

PEERS

TEENS CARE AN enormous amount about what their friends and classmates think of them. Even the most independent and free-thinking adolescent wants the respect of his or her peers; it is simply human nature. Most teens like to conform, blend in, and not make any waves. Until recently, most people saw vegetarianism as a fringe movement, one that attracted people who "hugged trees and ate loads of granola." These stereotypes have never been true, as you have already read, but they persisted until recently in American high schools and colleges. Now, as more and more teens are becoming vegetarians, attitudes are changing, but do not be surprised if you are harassed by your peers for choosing a meatless diet.

LIFE AT SCHOOL

The classroom is one place where teasing can get out of control, as high-schooler Susan Thomas can attest: "I once asked to be excused from biology because we were dissecting frogs and I refused to do that. When I got back, some other students had put all their frog parts in my bag." Fellow students can be pretty insensitive, thinking that practical jokes are no big deal, whereas, in fact, if the jokers get out of hand, they can make life pretty hard for their vegetarian classmates.

The best thing is to ignore immature behavior and try to remain open-minded about people's attitudes. If other kids confront you directly about your choice, you can either tell them that what you eat is your business, or better still, offer to explain some of your reasons. You should have no problem getting materials together to show people, as there are literally hundreds of books, magazine and newspaper articles, and even scientific reports on the benefits of vegetarianism.

Claire Adams tells of when she and her sister Elana were harassed at school: "People used to tease us at school. They would wave meat in our faces. . . . They would also joke about how pale and unhealthy we would look. We didn't have any friends who were vegetarians and no one really understood." Elana adds, "Going to restaurants with friends can be weird. If you're at a huge table of twenty and all your friends order meat and you get a salad, it just looks weird. I remember people joking that all we ate was lettuce." The two sisters were happy they had each other and their firm belief that what they were doing was right.

Mike Ravitz also encountered opposition from his peers when he announced he was a vegetarian. "At first when I became a vegetarian, I would get into heated arguments with my friends. They would taunt me and it would escalate and I thought, 'This isn't working.'" Mike decided not to "publish" the fact that he had chosen a vegan diet and that he would explain it to people only when they asked.

WHEN PEOPLE THINK YOU ARE WEIRD

Besides suffering in biology class, Susan Thomas admits that it is hard to know that people sometimes think you are strange. "People think it's really weird. One girl was making fun of me because of my 'religion' and I said, 'It's not my religion, it's my choice.'" Susan found it very hard to enlighten people at her high school and hopes that at college she will find more like-minded peers.

FLAWS IN YOUR ARGUMENT

Some teenage vegetarians find it hard to answer questions like, "How can you call yourself a vegetarian when you still wear leather?" As we have discussed, there are several types of vegetarians in the world and everyone's definition is a little different. Nevertheless, if you are caught off guard, it is hard to make a coherent argument on the spot with someone who is looking to argue.

Teen Danielle Pierce had to navigate her way through some difficult situations at school. She explains,

There were some people at my school . . . who would ask me all kinds of questions, trying to get me to crack. If people asked me why I was a vegetarian and I said for ethical reasons, I didn't feel that I could explain clearly to them without getting nervous because I knew they were waiting for me to slip up. After a year or so, when I was educated about the whole picture, I felt really good about it and I could defend myself coherently. I didn't feel that I needed to convert them, but I felt good that I could explain to the people who were really pressuring me. Education is the only way to overcome that.

Danielle became the head of both the ecology club and the ethical treatment for animals club. She organized presentations about the environment and vegetarianism, handed out literature on both subjects, and took part in conferences for teens. "I thought that even if people didn't agree with my reasons and beliefs," she says, "I could at least try to raise some awareness about the issues."

Sometimes it is difficult for teens to deal with the perceived contradictions in anything less than a "total" vegetarian diet. Jenny Orvis says, "A couple of months ago, a classmate confronted me about wearing leather and being a vegetarian. I explained it was difficult to reconcile, it's why I don't protest anymore, but in my heart, I still feel bad about it." Remember the words of artist and activist Sue Coe: "You're doing the best you can."

Claire Adams had a similar experience. "Once at school I was having a conversation about vegetarianism and animal rights with someone and then he looked down at my shoes and I just felt so embarrassed and ridiculous. It wasn't so much that I cared what the other person thought, but here I am defending animals, going on and on about how they shouldn't be killed, and there I was wearing leather shoes." Claire feels that it's just too hard to find nice nonleather shoes, but she hopes to give up leather in the future.

As a teenager you have a lot to think about; vegetarianism adds a whole new dimension that requires time, energy, sacrifice, and patience. To whatever degree you decide to extend your vegetarianism is entirely your business and you have absolutely no obligation to anyone to explain yourself. If someone calls you a hypocrite for wearing leather or feathers and calling yourself a vegetarian, tell them life is more complicated than that.

Hopefully you have not chosen vegetarianism to win a popularity contest. You want to stop eating meat and perhaps eliminate other animal products from your life for many of the reasons already discussed in this book. People, especially teenagers, often tease and harass other teens regarding beliefs and practices about which the teasers know little or nothing. Sometimes you just encounter bullies or people who think they will be more popular with a group if they pick on you for being different. Be true to your convictions; know that you are doing something good for yourself, for animals, and for the environment; and seek support from other vegetarians.

WHAT TO DO WHEN EATING OUT

GOING OUT TO eat is a great American tradition and an excellent way to get together with family and friends. If you are a vegetarian, you may feel that you are limited to green salads or spaghetti with butter or tomato sauce. Fortunately, more restaurants in all parts of the country have started offering vegetarian options from out-of-the-ordinary pastas to exotic stir-fries. Melissa Smith admits, "When I go out with my friends and they say, 'Let's get a burger,' I have to say no. But now I have all kinds of options to choose from."

If you are concerned that there will be nothing on the menu for you to eat, you can do a number of things. You can call the restaurant and ask if they have any vegetarian options. If they say no, you can always ask if the chef might prepare you a simple meal from vegetables and rice, staples in most restaurant kitchens. Lisa Ravitz, Mike's mother, says, "We have been to some restaurants where the chef obviously saw us as a challenge and created some really wonderful things. We've also had the situation where we've been given a plate of half-raw vegetables." In a worst-case scenario, if the restaurant has absolutely nothing you can eat, you can always bring your own food. If the establishment protests, suggest that perhaps they add one or two vegetarian options. Remember to be polite and perhaps have your parents explain the situation. To avoid a scene, no matter how small, it is always a good idea to call ahead.

THE FAST-FOOD DILEMMA

A lot of teens do most of their away-from-home dining in fast-food restaurants, such as McDonald's and Burger King. The main staple at these places is the hamburger, but they are slowly beginning to offer other choices. The corporations that run these restaurants know that vegetarianism is popular with teenagers right now and are developing ways to feed them what they want. You can always order a hamburger with all the fixings, asking that they just hold the burger. Many places offer salads, and establishments like Taco Bell have vegetarian tacos and burritos. If you are only a no-red-meat vegetarian, then chicken and fish sandwiches are options for you. You do not have to say no every time the gang wants to go to Wendy's. However, while there are an increasing number of alternatives for you at fast-food restaurants, they are still not the best choices. Fast food tends to be relatively high in calories and fat for the nutritional value it provides. Next time your friends want to go to a fast-food restaurant, suggest a healthier snack alternative such as frozen yogurt, bagels, or even pizza.

I STILL GET EMBARRASSED

Marcie Welsh knows there are many options for vegetarians dining out these days, but it can still be difficult at times. "If there is a place that everyone wants to go to and there is just nothing for me to eat, I have to say no. People would sometimes roll their eyes and feel they have to change their plans. I get a little embarrassed at times." When you decide to become a vegetarian, eating out is one of the added challenges you will face. Some situations will be uncomfortable, but with a little planning, restaurants can generally accommodate everyone.

HOW TO MANAGE THE SCHOOL CAFETERIA

LUNCHTIME AT SCHOOL can be anything from a quick bite of cafeteria chow between classes to a leisurely meal shared with friends. A number of vegetarian teens bring their lunch from home so they do not have to worry about what the kitchen is serving up. However, as the number of vegetarian teens grows, so too do their options. Matthew Brewi, chef at Berkeley-Carroll School in Brooklyn, New York, says, "I realized there were a number of students who were vegetarians and asked them what they might like to eat." Brewi now includes at least one vegetarian option each day, complemented by a salad bar. "The response has been very positive and we're always looking for ways to improve and diversify the menus."

One of the best tools to have if you want your high school or college food service to regularly serve good vegetarian food is the *Healthy School Lunch Action Guide*, written by Susan Campbell and Todd Winant. Schools across the country have used the guide as a "road map" to creating successful and popular programs that get kids interested in eating balanced and wholesome meals during the day. Suggest the manual to your school administrator or food service director and tell them that it offers:

- ◇ Ways to present healthy meals in an appealing fashion
- ◇ Methods for educating others on the benefits of healthy eating
- ◇ Teaching aids, lesson plans, activities, handouts, letters, curriculum ideas, and lists of affiliated organizations
- ◇ A detailed list explaining why eating a healthier diet not only benefits us, but the environment and the rest of the world
- ◇ Recipes, food preparation guidelines, and nutritional information

Creating more nutritious and socially responsible meals at your school is a team effort, one that should include your parents, friends, educators, and school chefs. If your school does not seem receptive to the idea of healthier lunches, call the Healthy School Lunch Program at EarthSave (listed in Chapter 7 under "Organizations"); they can offer useful advice.

WHAT TO EAT AT OTHER PEOPLE'S HOUSES

MANY TEENS ARE nervous that when they go to a friend's house for dinner there will be nothing for them to eat. How do they ask politely for a vegetarian option? Elana Adams says, "My mother used to call ahead and discuss the issue with my friend's mother or father." Most of the time, she says, they made something like pasta or a big salad for Elana to eat. By calling ahead, you can also offer to bring something of your own, like a veggie burger or some rice and beans from last night's dinner at home. If someone is having a party or a special birthday dinner, ask if there is anything you can do to help and again, offer to bring at least part of the meal for yourself. As Marcie Welsh admits, "If people are making a fancy meal, they feel bad if they can't do something to feed you the same way. When I bring food for myself, it takes some of the pressure off."

If you are having a spontaneous meal at someone's house, ask politely if they have anything in the refrigerator or cupboard that you could possibly eat. You may have to be willing to eat something that is not your favorite food.

HOW TO GET THROUGH THE HOLIDAYS

THE NUMBER ONE activity at most holiday gatherings is eating. When people think of Thanksgiving, Passover, or Christmas, for example, the first thing that usually comes to mind is a big meal with delicious food. These meals generally center on a large piece of meat or fowl, with many side dishes to complement the main course. If you are a vegetarian, holidays can be a stressful time when it comes to "the big meal." As Jenny Orvis says, "My first big fight with my parents about being a vegetarian was when I wouldn't eat turkey at Thanksgiving."

One way to handle holidays, whether you are at home or going to a relative's house, is, again, to take responsibility for what you are going to eat. Most meals consist of several side dishes that offer more than adequate nutritional value, like sweet potatoes, stuffing (not cooked in the turkey), salad, and rice dishes. If you or your parents are concerned you still will not have enough, bring along a veggie or soy patty as a main course. Your relatives will probably ask if you wish you could have some juicy white meat instead of your nut loaf. Remind them that you are abstaining from meat by choice, and that no one is forcing you not to take a slice of turkey.

HOW TO WORK AROUND RELIGIOUS CEREMONIES

AS WITH HOLIDAYS, religious ceremonies, such as confirmations and bar mitzvahs, are often a time when family and friends gather together and share a large meal. Many religions have rules about what people can and cannot eat; for example, pork is forbidden in strict Islamic and Jewish households, while beef is not permitted in certain Hindu homes. If Easter is a time to share lamb with your relations, than simply make or bring an alternative. During a Passover seder, the holiday meal and ceremony, some of the rituals involve eating eggs, and meat is usually served as a main course. If you come from a very religious home, some relatives may be offended by your abstinence. Try to explain before the ceremony why you do not eat meat so as to avoid a scene in the middle of dinner.

Mike Ravitz's mother, Lisa, says that certain Jewish holidays, such as Rosh Hashanah, involve the use of honey, which Mike will not eat as a vegan. "My mom thinks I'm missing out because I don't taste the sweetness of the honey, but I feel much better knowing that I didn't kill any bees to taste that sweetness." The hard part of navigating dietary restrictions and religious ceremonies is remaining true to yourself while, ideally, not offending anyone. You know your family better than anyone else, so figure out the best way to discuss the issue long before it might become a problem.

WHEN YOU ARE TRAVELING

TRYING NEW TASTES and flavors when you are away from home is one of the most exciting aspects of traveling. As a vegetarian there are many options open to you, especially in cultures that use vegetables and grains as their main sources of food rather than meat. These cultures include most of China, India, Africa, and Central and South America. If you are vacationing in the United States or Europe, you are far more likely to run into meat-centered meals. There are several ways that you and your family can have a relaxing trip without worrying about your vegetarian requirements. Some ways to make the journey easier include the following:

◇ Airlines will serve you a vegetarian meal if you call ahead and order one. Once you are on the plane, the flight attendant will probably serve you first, which is another benefit.

◇ Call ahead and ask the hotel where you are staying if they have vegetarian meals in their restaurants or at least a well-stocked salad bar.

◇ Most guidebooks have extensive lists of restaurants and what type of food they offer. Plan which ones you want to go to before you leave home. If you have any questions, you can always call them.

◇ Bring along as many nutritious snacks as you can while traveling as long as you can carry them and they will not spoil too rapidly.

◇ Remind your parents that you will be flexible if need be. They want to know that you will eat *something* if there are absolutely no other options.

Claire Adams says, "We spent most of my childhood traveling around Europe, the United States, and Mexico, and both my sister and I were vegetarians. I can't remember ever not being able to find something, somewhere to eat." As with most aspects of vegetarianism, it just might take a little extra work.

IF YOU ARE ON A DATE

DATING MAKES MOST people nervous. What am I going to wear? Does my hair look funny? What will we eat? This last question can cause you particular angst if you are a vegetarian. You know why you have chosen your diet and have all the reasons lined up neatly in your mind, but you still may fear rejection from a date because you do not eat meat. What if your partner thinks vegetarians are weird? Well, a date is a perfect opportunity to prove him or her wrong.

Claire Adams remembers having boyfriends who threatened to "dump me if I didn't stop being a vegetarian. They thought it wasn't cool." Claire, who has been a vegetarian since she was a child, has since decided not to date anyone who does not understand why she is a vegetarian. Jenny Orvis says she has never been confronted by a date, but that if she were, "I'd let him know why I don't eat meat and hopefully educate him about the issues."

One good way to avoid an uncomfortable scene is to make sure you are going to a restaurant that prepares both vegetarian and nonvegetarian food. If your date does not know you do not eat meat, and does not figure it out by what you are eating, it is up to you to tell him or her if you choose. If you do not think you want to see the person again, you can avoid the issue entirely. However, if you do want to continue seeing the person, a discussion of your diet is a pretty good idea.

WHEN YOU ARE AT CAMP

CAMP, LIKE SCHOOL, is a place where chefs make large amounts of food for big groups of people. Because they are cooking on such a large scale, it is not always so easy to prepare food for special diets. If you are going to sleep-away camp, have your parents call the camp director and discuss what options are available for a vegetarian. Most of the time, there is enough to eat, but see whether tofu can be added to the list of items at a salad bar or as one of the main dishes a few nights a week.

Many camps have been keeping up with the times. Jenny Orvis says, "When I went away to sleep-away camp at age 9, there were only a couple of vegetarians; they had maybe one dish for us. Three years later they had a whole table of choices because so many people had become vegetarians." When there were barbecues at Mike Ravitz's camp, he would eat one of the veggie burgers that he brought from home and kept in the camp freezer. "If anyone asked what I was eating," he says, "I would explain that I was a vegan and what that was, but I did not advertise the fact that I was a vegetarian."

SPORTS AND VEGETARIANISM

SPORTS ARE A very important component to teen life. Whether you are on a varsity team at school or you just enjoy running a few miles a week around your neighborhood, physical exercise is important to you. Most parents, and many teens, worry that, as vegetarians, they will not have enough energy for athletics. This is simply not true as evidenced by all the famous athletes who are both record-breakers and vegetarians, including Dave Scott, long considered the world's greatest triathlete, and Sixto Linares, world-record holder for the longest single-day triathlon. Sixto remarks, "[W]hen I became a vegetarian in high school, my parents were very very upset that I wouldn't eat meat . . . After fourteen years, they are finally accepting that it's good for me. They know it's not going to kill me."[1] At first Sixto was a lacto-ovo vegetarian, but he has since slowly removed eggs and dairy from his diet.

Your parents may be concerned about sports and vegetarianism, but assure them that you will discuss your diet with your doctor, school health professional, and/or coach to determine a healthy plan. You may simply have to increase your caloric intake to match the calories that you burn while exercising. Remember that it is not more protein you need while doing hard physical work, but carbohydrates, our real source of energy. As a strict vegetarian through high school, I had no trouble running long-distance races and playing lacrosse, as well as hiking, skiing, kayaking, and mountain biking.

WHY SUPPORT IS SO IMPORTANT

WHEN YOU BECOME a vegetarian, some moments are easier than others. You may get tired of answering questions about your beliefs and what you eat. You may also find it particularly difficult to deal with teasing and insensitive comments from family, friends, and even strangers. Susan Thomas comments, "Sometimes people are going to give you a hard time, so joining a group can be very helpful." As more and more teens choose vegetarianism, the support network for them has grown tremendously. Both national and local vegetarian groups and organizations are ideal resources for learning how to cope, finding out nutritional information, and understanding why your parents may be so angry about your new diet plans.

GROUPS

Sally Clinton, founder of the Vegetarian Education Network (VEN), says that when she became a vegetarian, "there weren't many groups out there." Now that so many teens are vegetarians, she thinks "young people definitely need support. It's very difficult growing up in a meat-based culture, where so much is against vegetarianism. I think it's very important to have a support network and that's what I tried to provide by starting the Vegetarian Education Network." VEN runs groups, seminars, and trips for teens who are interested in a vegetarian lifestyle and sound ecological living.

Nutritionist Brenda Davis, whose kids are vegetarians, feels that it is also very important for teens to find support. "Groups that can be specifically geared towards teens," she says, "like VEN, Youth for Environmental Sanity (YES), EarthSave, and People for the Ethical Treatment of Animals

(PETA), help teens become educated so when people do question them, they can respond in an educated and confident way. They can demonstrate that this wasn't a decision based on a whim, but one based on serious thought."

LENDING A HAND

If you want to learn more about vegetarianism and get in contact with other vegetarians, volunteering for a national organization or one in your high school is a good way. Susan Thomas says, "Working for VEN and their magazine, *How on Earth*, has helped me a lot because I realize there are people out there who believe what I believe even if they aren't in my community." Danielle Pierce also works for VEN and says, "Working for VEN is fantastic because not only do I learn something new every day about vegetarian and ecological issues, but I also get to help others understand. A lot of parents call and have questions about their kids. I get to calm them down." You can use the resources provided in Chapter 7 to help you get in touch with such groups and become an advocate for vegetarianism.

I'M NOT ALONE

"Groups are important," says Jenny Orvis, "because they make me feel like I'm not alone." When you become involved with an organization, you come into contact with anywhere from a few dozen to thousands of other teenage vegetarians who have probably gone through a lot of what you are experiencing and feeling. You can hear how someone handled not eating turkey at Thanksgiving or how another person went from lacto-ovo vegetarianism to veganism.

Mike Ravitz attended a weeklong program called Animal

Learn sponsored by the American Anti-Vivisection League with other vegetarians. "I learned all about vegetarianism and after a week, I decided to give strict vegetarianism a shot. Since then, I've kept with it." He adds, "Knowing a lot and that there are others has helped me stick with it. Since that summer, I've kept active with what they're doing. The leader of the league has come to my school several times and we've had wonderful discussions."

SUPPORT AT SCHOOL

Your school is one of the best places to find other vegetarians to discuss issues that concern you. If your school does not have a vegetarian or ecology club, then start one. Ask your school administrator how to begin and then ask your friends to help get the club going. Mike Ravitz says, "I'm an active member of an animal rights club at my school. What we've done in the club is say that we're not going to criticize anyone. We try to educate everyone about the facts, good and bad, and let them know they can be as active a member as they want to be. That's our philosophy and so far it's been very successful."

Danielle Pierce says, "Involvement at school is so important. It's the only thing that kept me going because there was really very little awareness. I would encourage everyone to get involved at school. It really helps."

A LITTLE HELP FROM MY FRIENDS

Most teens learn about vegetarianism from their friends. They can feel intimidated by large groups and not want to seek support from a national or even school organization. In this case, as well as others, your vegetarian friends are the best source you can use. "A lot of my friends are vegetarians," says Marcie Welsh. "We often get together and figure out fun recipes and new foods to try." Whether you want to find out which fast-food restaurants, if any, serve vegetarian food, or you just need someone to talk to about how difficult it is planning meals with your parents, try your friends and see what advice they have to offer. You may even make some new vegetarian friends along the way.

VEGETARIAN DIPLOMACY

THE MORE YOU get caught up in vegetarianism and its growing popularity, the more you may feel that *everyone* should feel the same enthusiasm. It is important to remember that while the horrors of the meat and dairy industries and the health benefits of a vegetarian diet are enough to convince *you* to give up meat, they may not convince everyone. As artist Sue Coe states, "People don't become vegetarians by force. It has to happen through education." In fact, you may end up actually discouraging some people from trying vegetarianism if you are too pushy.

Young people have a lot to say on the subject of vegetarianism and converting the world. Every vegetarian teen has had to decide how best to handle explaining his or her vegetarianism without seeming preachy. Some think that unless everyone does as they do, we are all doomed. Thankfully, most teens have come to the conclusion that teaching by example is the best way to be a vegetarian and to not alienate others. Mike Ravitz says,

> I'll leave other people alone, just like I want to be left alone. I feel I can do more by keeping to myself than possibly turning someone off vegetarianism. I once went on a summer program for two months and

no one knew I was a vegetarian until the end. I don't make it a public issue. If someone is curious and asks, I'm more than happy to discuss vegetarianism, but I don't think you get much accomplished if you're forceful.

Claire Adams says, "The way to really prove a point is to do something on a daily basis, as an individual, using yourself as an example, rather than by pressuring people." Claire has also said that she finds it "incomprehensible" that people eat meat, but has learned that to some extent what an individual eats is his or her business. Susan Thomas advises not "really advertising the fact you're a vegetarian at first. Just by being quiet, people are more likely to follow your example."

One of the hardest issues that both vegetarian and nonvegetarian teens must face is that of being judged. Every day they may feel that not only are their parents and teachers judging them, but their friends and classmates too. As a vegetarian, you will encounter many people who will be quick to judge you solely based on the fact that you do not eat meat. It is best to stay calm when this happens and try to explain yourself or remind people that what you eat is your business. Jenny Orvis states, "I try not to judge others because I know that certain things I do are hypocritical. It's hard to stand in someone else's shoes and make their decisions for them."

Similarly, although you've made the decision to be a vegetarian, you should not judge those who eat meat. Marcie Welsh sums it up nicely: "I think you can encourage people to be vegetarians, but you can't force them. You can tell them the reasons, but to say that everyone should be a vegetarian just doesn't work." Coming to their own conclusions, without pressure from adults, is what most adolescents want. Vegetarian teens tend to be particularly aware of this and usually live their lives accordingly.

A JUGGLING ACT

YOU LEAD A very busy life, and putting it all together is an ongoing challenge. Incorporating vegetarianism into this crowded roster often adds new dimensions, concerns, and difficulties. If you take it slowly, learn as much as you can, and seek support when you need it, you will begin to forget what life was like before you were a vegetarian. It will become second nature.

One way to make your life easier as a vegetarian is to know what elements go into a balanced diet. The next chapter focuses on all the nutritional information you need to know in order to be healthy. There is much to learn, but again, after a short while, you will be an authority on subjects like alternate protein sources and calcium-rich vegetables.

5

EVERYTHING YOU NEED TO KNOW
ABOUT NUTRITION

I think there needs to be a greater push for more nutritional information for teens so they can make informed decisions. They should know everything they can.

—Dakota Prosch, teenage vegetarian

MOST teens do not want to think too much about what they have to eat to maintain good health. Honestly, most adults do not want to think about it either. As a vegetarian you probably will have to pay a little more attention to what you are consuming each day, but you certainly do not have to focus all of your attention on meal planning. There are a few basic nutritional points to keep in mind:

◇ Do not replace foods that you have taken out of your diet with "empty" calories from things high in fat and sugar. Parents are most concerned that when teens stop eating animal products, they will eat only french fries and potato chips.

◇ Do not eat too much of any one thing at each meal. Try to balance your nutrients over the course of the day.

◇ Use your body as a guide. If you are feeling sluggish or cannot concentrate during the day, try having a healthy snack of dried fruit, carrot sticks, or some rice cakes with peanut butter for a quick pick-me-up.

In general, you should eat the following each day:

- ◆6 or more servings of whole grains each day, including bread, pasta, and rice
- ◆3–5 servings of vegetables daily
- ◆2–3 servings of beans, nuts, seeds, and a meat alternative— for example, tofu or textured vegetable protein (TVP)
- ◆3 or more servings of fruit during the day
- ◆6 to 8 servings of milk or a milk alternative each day; alternatives include soy, rice, and almond milk

A word about fat: Although many people think fat is bad, the truth is that we need fat in our diet. However, it is best to keep your fat intake to less than 30 percent of your total calorie intake; some research recommends less than 20 percent or even less than 10 percent. But some fat sources are better than others. Saturated fats—those found in butter, meat, cheese—are the least healthy. A better choice is the unsaturated fats found in canola and olive oils, nuts, and olives.

If you ever have a question about nutrition and are not sure what to do, consult one of the many guides, books, or journals published specifically for vegetarian health, or ask your doctor to put you in touch with a nutritionist who specializes in vegetarianism.

NUTRITIONAL HOT SPOTS

YOUR BODY NEEDS certain nutrients each day to maintain good health. During the teen years, when you nearly double your body weight, your nutritional requirements are pretty much at their height. Parents are often hysterical, worried that their vegetarian teenager will be protein deficient, get scurvy, or die before he or she reaches the next birthday. The truth is, nutrition is fairly simple: If you eat enough calories from the right foods, you will have more than enough energy to get through the day. In addition, if you keep your diet reasonably balanced, you will likely be healthier than you were before you became a vegetarian.

In this chapter, you will learn helpful information about the following:

◇Calories

◇Carbohydrates

◇Fats

◇Protein

◇Calcium

◇Iron

◇Zinc

◇Fiber

◇Vitamin B-12

◇Vitamin C

◇Vitamin D

Certain nutrients are more difficult to acquire in a vegan diet than in a lacto-ovo diet simply because you are eating fewer things. If you are a vegan, for example, and you are concerned about B-12, daily supplements are available and you should take them. I recommend that if you are now or plan to become a vegan, you should take a daily supplement to ensure that you are getting all the vitamins and minerals your rapidly growing body needs. Do not forget to consult someone about which supplements you may need.

CALORIES

You have probably heard the term *calories* quite a lot and are not quite sure exactly what they are or why they are so important. They are essentially a measurement of heat—more precisely, how much heat it takes to raise the temperature of a kilogram of water one degree Celsius. Our bodies use calories from food as energy for all of our systems. As a teen, you need about 50 percent more calories for good nutrition than you will as an adult because you are growing so fast. Unfortunately, American teenagers tend to eat too many calories, do not exercise enough, and are often overweight. However, if you need to gain weight or need more energy during the day, try adding trail mix, milk shakes, and dried fruits to your diet.

We all need calories and most foods have them (water is one of the very few substances that does not), but we do not use all calories the same way. We need nutrients that are provided by a variety of foods. Generally, if you are getting enough calories during the day from a balanced diet, then you are getting enough nutrients. But the key is *balance*; your calories have to come from the variety of food groups listed earlier, not exclusively from one category. In other words, 2,000 calories from a combination of protein, carbohydrates, fruits, vegetables, dairy products, and some essential fats will keep you healthy and strong: 2,000 calories' worth of cupcakes will not.

CARBOHYDRATES

Carbohydrates, which certainly contain calories, are what we use for energy and they burn very efficiently as fuel. When you do vigorous, heart-pounding exercise, you use a lot of calories from carbohydrates. Teens tend to be very active and have high requirements for this nutrient in their diets. Vegetables such as potatoes, yams, and corn are good sources of complex carbohydrates, as are other starches like breads, grains, pasta, and brown rice. Because so many of our daily calories should come from carbohydrates, it is important to make sure you are eating enough of them.

You may think you are limited by the grains and breads you see in the supermarket, but one trip to a health food or Middle Eastern store, if there is one near you, will introduce you to more exotic grains like couscous, amaranth, and quinoa, as well as several varieties of whole-grain breads. Try to stay away from foods such as white rice and products made from white flour and/or white sugar, as manufacturers generally process out most of the nutritive value of these foods.

FATS

A lot of people, including teens, think that it is best to avoid fat in their diets, especially if they are trying to lose weight. While it is important not to eat too many fatty foods, such as french fries and cheese, you still need some fat in your daily diet. On a daily basis, we burn some fat as energy and also store it in our fatty tissue. As teenagers, boys usually gain more muscle mass than girls, who tend to simply gain more fat. No two teenagers will put on weight the same so try not to compare yourself to other people who appear to eat whatever they want and never gain weight.

All fat is not created equally and, happily, the saturated fat that you stop eating when you give up meat and other animal products is the worst for you. Saturated fat is more harmful to your health, raises your blood cholesterol level, and leads to heart disease more often than does unsaturated fat. As we have discussed, most people think that heart disease is an affliction of the elderly, but studies performed on young people show that the first evidence of fatty deposits in the coronary arteries shows up as early as age 3.

Though simply being a vegetarian will help reduce fat generally, and saturated fat specifically, the best solution is to limit your fat intake to anywhere between 20 to 30 percent of the calories you eat each day (some scientists even believe 10 percent). Healthier alternatives to foods that contain saturated fats, such as butter, meat, and cheese, include vegetable oils, such as olive and canola; avocado; and nut butters, such as peanut and almond.

Vegetable fats are better for you in terms of heart disease and cancer, but they are still fat. The best plan is to keep fatty foods to a minimum in your diet now so you will not suffer their effects in the future.

PROTEIN

If you are a vegetarian, there is one question you will hear over and over again from people young and old: "How do you get enough protein?" There are so many myths about protein that it is difficult to debunk them all. Some of them are:

◇ *Vegetarians do not get enough protein.* The truth is that most Americans eat way too much protein and need much less in their diets than they imagine.

◇ *The only good sources of protein are meat and dairy products.* In fact, vegetables have enough protein to supply anyone's needs and they are much less harmful in terms of fat, hormones, and other harmful by-products. You have to eat more vegetables than you would meat, but then you are also getting more of other nutrients, such as calcium and zinc.

◆ *To get a full complement of the eight daily essential amino acids, which are the building blocks of protein, you need to eat foods in certain combinations—for example, rice and beans.* This idea was long held as the way for vegetarians to get "complete" proteins, but now scientists believe that if you eat certain protein-rich foods on their own, over the course of the day, that is enough.

◆ *The only available protein sources for vegetarians are tofu and peanut butter.* Not true; the Food and Nutrition Board recommends that 10 percent of your daily calories come from protein. Many plants have much more than this figure, and broccoli and kale each have about 45 percent protein for their calories. Most vegetables contain somewhere between 15 and 45 percent of their calories from protein. Excellent sources of protein include dark leafy greens, all cabbage-family vegetables, fresh beans and peas, sprouts, soy products, meat analogues (such as textured vegetable protein), seeds, grains, and nuts. Eggs and cheese are also good protein foods if you eat them.

The experts tend to agree that if you get enough calories each day, then do not worry; you are more than likely getting enough protein. In fact, you will be much healthier because some of the latest studies indicate that too much protein, particularly animal protein, contributes to all of the diseases we have already discussed, such as cancer, heart disease, and diabetes. The foods that do not contain much protein are fruits, fats, and sugars, so do not base your diet on these substances alone.

PLANT PROTEINS ARE HEALTHIER We know you can certainly get enough protein from plants. An added benefit is that protein from plants is better for you because they generally contain less fat, have no cholesterol, lower your blood cholesterol levels, and do not promote loss of calcium from bones. You can eat far more vegetables without worrying about fat and calories than you can meat. Meat tends to make people feel full in an uncomfortable, stuffed way. Your digestive system is more efficient at working with vegetable matter and moves it along more quickly, so you generally do not have the same heavy feeling associated with meat.

WHAT'S THE BIG DEAL? You may wonder why people make such a fuss about protein anyway. Why do we need protein in our diets? Protein plays a major role in building, repairing, and maintaining our bodies, so it is essential that we get enough of it. As you touch your hair, feel your bones, and look at all the different components of your body, remember that almost every part is made up of protein. Proteins consist of substances called amino acids, eight of which we call *essential amino acids* because we need them every day. They are:

> ◇ Tryptophan
>
> ◇ Phenylalanine
>
> ◇ Leucine
>
> ◇ Isoleucine
>
> ◇ Lysine
>
> ◇ Valine

◇Methionine

◇Threonine

These eight are found in all plant foods, along with the other nonessential fourteen, in different ratios.

WHAT EXACTLY ARE MY PROTEIN NEEDS?

Everyone's nutritional needs vary depending on a number of factors, such as age, weight, gender, and activity level. However, there are some guidelines you can follow that will give you a good idea of how much protein you need to consume each day.

Girls and Women		Boys and Men	
11 to 18 years:	46 grams	11 to 14 years:	45 grams
19 to 51 years:	44 grams	15 to 51 years:	56 grams

Do not worry if you are not getting exactly these amounts. As we have stated: *Enough calories equals enough protein.*

CALCIUM

Calcium is very important for maintaining our bones and keeping our hearts beating, our diaphragms moving, and all of our other muscles contracting. Our need for it is never greater than during adolescence and it is very important that teens have good sources of calcium. Most people think that milk is the best source of calcium, but as we have discussed earlier, milk and dairy products are not necessarily the best providers, and they contain a lot of fat and by-products. Dairy products are also low in iron, a problem for teenage girls, and should not be relied on as a primary source of calcium. Try a soy milk fortified with calcium or plants such as kale, beans, and broccoli, which are naturally rich in the substance.

Here are a few important things you should know about calcium:

◇ Health experts disagree as to how much calcium a teenager needs, but most assert that somewhere between 1,200 and 1,600 milligrams is about right.

◇ Calcium needs vary, but some studies show that vegetarians do not need to take in as much because they lose less through their blood than meat eaters.

◇ Some experts think that young women should not drink soda, which contains phosphorus. The phosphorus flushes calcium out of the system through the feces. Young women need calcium in greater amounts than do young men.

◇ Your bone density, which is determined during adolescence and young adulthood, is dependent not only on calcium for good health, but also on physical activity—so exercise regularly!

◇ Good sources of calcium include tofu (processed with calcium sulfate), sesame butter, collard greens, mustard greens, kale, broccoli, cabbage, brussels sprouts, most beans, dried fruits, figs, seeds, and fortified soy milk and orange juice.

It may take a little while to remember all the new and varied sources of calcium, especially if you've been dependent on dairy products. However, in practically no time you'll be wondering why you ever drank so much milk in the first place.

Calcium is vital to everyone's health, especially teens. Teenage vegans may find it hard to maintain an adequate supply and therefore should take a calcium supplement of some kind.

IRON

For healthy blood, you need iron, and as a teenager, your daily requirements are pretty high. This is especially true for girls, who lose a lot of iron through menstruation. Most parents think that the best source of iron is red meat, but plenty of plant sources provide ample amounts. You will also avoid all the fat, cholesterol, and quite often hormones and antibiotics if you do not eat meat.

Some good tips about iron are as follows:

◇ You will absorb the most iron if you eat it in conjunction with a vitamin C–rich food, such as orange juice or broccoli.

◇ Dairy products inhibit the absorption of iron.

◇ Girls need more iron than boys. Girls need about 15 milligrams each day, whereas boys need only about 12 milligrams. Vegetarian girls should take an iron supplement each day.

◇ An abundance of iron is found in broccoli, raisins, chickpeas, spinach, watermelon, blackstrap molasses, pinto beans, black-eyed peas, lentils, bran flakes, and fortified cereals.

◇ If you cook food in a cast-iron skillet or other iron pots, you can actually increase your iron intake.

You should include iron in your vegetarian diet every day. If people try to tell you that the only way to get iron is by eating beef and pork, have your list of alternatives ready.

ZINC

Zinc is necessary for both normal growth and sexual maturation; in addition, it plays a central role in how your immune system responds. If you are seriously zinc deficient, your wounds do not heal, you can have nervous disorders, and your senses of smell and taste can be impaired. These disorders are not common and it is easy to get enough of this mineral in your diet by eating legumes such as black-eyed peas and refried beans, oatmeal, bran flakes, nuts, pumpkin, mushrooms, green peas, asparagus, dark leafy vegetables, nutritional yeast (as opposed to baker's yeast), and some whole grains. Milk and soy milk are also good sources of zinc.

Formerly, scientists thought that zinc was best absorbed from meat, but now believe that high levels of both protein and phosphorus may raise your needs for the mineral. In any case, you should make sure to eat enough zinc-rich foods each day to ensure healthy levels.

FIBER

If the first thing that comes to your mind when you hear the word *fiber* is oat bran, think again. Proper amounts of fiber in your diet are necessary to protect the digestive system, maintain healthy blood vessels, and ensure regular elimination. Fiber, which is found only in plant foods, also helps your immune system fight disease, lowers the risk of both cancer and heart disease, helps lower blood cholesterol, and assists in keeping diabetes under control.

On the whole, vegetarians eat more fiber than nonvegetarians. They consume anywhere from two to four times more than the average American, who eats about 12 grams each day. A balanced vegetarian diet is generally well stocked with fiber foods, including whole-wheat breads and rolls, beans, vegetables, fruits, rolled oats, and other grains.

While fiber is an important element in a vegetarian diet, it can inhibit the absorption of calcium, so you should avoid an excess amount of fiber in your diet.

VITAMIN B-12

Vitamin B-12 is by far the most hotly debated of all the vitamins in the vegetarian diet. Parents of vegans are very concerned about it because you can get B-12 only from eating animal products, and teens need 50 percent more of the vitamin than adults. Our need for vitamin B-12 is vital. It is necessary for proper nerve function, cell growth, and the prevention of anemia. If you were B-12 deficient, your skin would be hypersensitive, the surface of your tongue would become smooth, and you would experience nerve damage and fatigue. A deficiency of B-12 has terrible consequences, but it is rare; the actual amount we need is tiny.

If you are a lacto-ovo, lacto, or ovo vegetarian, you do not have to worry about the vitamin. We do store B-12 in our bodies for several years, but again, if you do not eat *any* animal products, look for a cereal fortified with the vitamin or take a vitamin supplement.

VITAMIN C

You will find vitamin C in an abundance of fruits and vegetables. They include:

◇Dark green leafy vegetables
◇Sweet peppers

◇Broccoli

◇Tomatoes

◇Cabbage-family vegetables

◇Berries

◇Citrus fruits

◇Asparagus

◇Fresh beans

◇Peas

◇Okra

◇Sprouts

Health experts believe that vitamin C helps prevent certain types of cancer, wards off infections, and aids the absorption of iron. It is also important for supporting cartilage, bone, teeth, and connective tissues in our bodies. As a vegetarian, your choices when it comes to vitamin C sources are both varied and usually easy to find.

VITAMIN D

Vitamin D, which is actually a hormone, is necessary for bone growth because it helps bones absorb calcium. One of the best sources of vitamin D is exposure to sunlight; most of us get enough daily to ensure healthy amounts. When your skin is exposed to sunlight, it produces vitamin D. Teenagers who have dark skin or live in cloudy or smoggy areas should take supplements to keep their vitamin D levels up. People who do not have enough vitamin D can develop a condition known as rickets, in which bones do not grow properly and become malformed. Your teeth, which are also dependent on calcium, may suffer if you are lacking in this vitamin.

Foods that have ample amounts of vitamin D include fish, milk, and eggs. If you are a vegan and spend time in the sun, your skin will produce enough of the vitamin. But remember, spending long periods of time in the sun is ultimately unhealthy for your skin. If you are a vegetarian other than vegan, try getting your vitamin D from dairy or eggs. If you are a vegan, take a multivitamin tablet. Also keep in mind that you do not want too much vitamin D because it becomes toxic above a certain level.

NAVIGATING VEGETARIAN NUTRITION

IT MAY SEEM like a lot to think about, but if you eat a properly balanced diet, and follow the guidelines given here, your nutritional requirements will be met. There are endless sources to help you find your way if you have questions; you should always feel free to ask your doctor or a nutritionist for advice. If you're not sure that their information is correct, as not all doctors or nutritionists are knowledgeable about vegetarianism specifically, do not give up. Continue your search until you come up with a satisfactory answer.

Before diving into the next chapter on how to prepare some delicious vegetarian dishes, I will present an extensive list of the nutritive benefits of many of the vegetables, fruits, grains, and nuts you will start to discover as a healthy vegetarian, as well as ways to prepare them.

TO BE HEALTHY, THAT IS THE ANSWER: HEALTH INFORMATION ABOUT VEGETABLES, FRUITS, GRAINS, AND NUTS

'Tis not the meat, but 'tis the appetite
Makes eating a delight.

—Sir John Suckling,
seventeenth-century English poet

VEGETABLES

Artichoke: **Health benefits:** Artichokes aid in the prevention of anemia, excessive acidity, diarrhea, rheumatism, bad breath, obesity, and glandular disorders.

Preparation tips: Steam until soft, then peel off leaves and dip in an oil-and-vinegar or vinaigrette dressing. Melted butter (if you eat dairy) or melted margarine also makes a nice dipping sauce. Scrape off leaf flesh with teeth. Continue to pick, peel, and eat until you reach the heart, often thought to be the best part, making sure to avoid the prickly nettles that come right before the heart.

Asparagus: **Health benefits:** Asparagus juice is purportedly good for rheumatism, neuritis, arthritis, and similar ailments.

Preparation tips: Tie asparagus spears in

bundles of about eight and boil in a pot with only the thick ends of the stalks in the water for about ten minutes. Flavor with a small amount of butter or lemon.

Carrot: **Health benefits:** Carrots, whole or as juice, are good for obesity, toxemia, constipation, asthma, poor complexion, poor teeth, insomnia, high blood pressure, and edema.

Preparation tips: Carrots are great raw, with or without skins. Use for dipping in guacamole or salsa. Eating them raw yields the most vitamins and nutrients. Shredded, they are good in slaws and salads. Try them in soups, mashed as a soufflé, or baked in the oven with honey.

Corn: **Health benefits:** Corn is good for cases of anemia, constipation, and emaciation.

Preparation tips: Some people like corn right off the cob, uncooked. Others prefer it steamed for three minutes and then sprinkled with a little salt and perhaps a trace of butter or margarine. Corn is very starchy and you should chew it thoroughly to ensure proper digestion. Other ways to make corn include roasted on a fire in its husk, off the cob in a salad, or in corn chowder.

Cucumber: **Health Benefits:** A natural diuretic, cucumbers promote the flow of urine and elimination of toxins from the body. They are also full of potassium, and are very good for both high and low blood pressure. Cucumbers also contain the enzyme erepsin, which aids in the digestion of proteins.

Preparation tips: Cucumbers are excellent in salads, used with dips, or by themselves. If you do not like the seeds, simply cut the cucumber lengthwise and scoop out the middle. Then cut whatever size slice you prefer.

Kale: **Health benefits:** With an enormous amount of vitamin A and calcium, kale is helpful with acidosis, constipation, obesity, poor teeth, arthritis, gout, skin diseases, and bladder disorders.

Preparation tips: Very good in salads, but be careful not eat too much, as it can produce gas. Boil in just enough water to cover the vegetable and cook for 25 to 35 minutes or until tender. Drain off water and season with salt, pepper, and butter or margarine.

Onion: **Health benefits:** Very good for clearing sinus infections. Onions are also good for healthy hair, nails, and eyes, and in cases of asthma and high blood pressure.

Preparation tips: Onions are used with many foods as a flavor enhancer. Stir-fries, stews, side dishes, entrées, salads, sauces, and breads all benefit from the addition of cooked or raw onions.

Peas: **Health benefits:** Peas are great for general nourishment and strengthening. They are good against anemia and help reduce blood cholesterol.

Preparation tips: You get the most benefit from eating peas raw. A great side vegetable, you can whip up a pot of peas with enough water to cover them and a little salt. Boil until tender. Peas are also very tasty in salads and stir-fries.

Spinach: **Health benefits:** Spinach is good for anemia, constipation, tumors, insomnia, obesity, high blood pressure, and bronchitis, among other things. Spinach has a lot of iron and you should eat it with foods high in vitamin C, such as oranges, to help with absorption.

Preparation tips: Eating spinach uncooked is the best way to enjoy its health benefits. When cooked, spinach causes the elimination of calcium from the bloodstream.

Sweet Potato: **Health benefits:** Full of vitamins and minerals, this holiday favorite is excellent if you need a lot of energy for hard physical labor. It is also good for stomach ulcers, hemorrhoids, and diarrhea.

Preparation tips: You can boil, bake, mash, cream, stew, or stuff sweet potatoes, adding pineapple, cinnamon, marshmallows, or anything else that sounds good to you. You can cook them with the skins or without, but an easy way to remove the outer layer is to first boil the potatoes for 20 to 30 minutes. The skin will then slip off easily.

Tomato: **Health benefits:** Tomatoes are natural antiseptics and protect against infections. If you eat a lot of tomatoes, they also improve your skin and purify your blood. Nicotinic acid in them helps reduce cholesterol and vitamin K can help prevent hemorrhages.

Preparation tips: As with sweet potatoes, tomatoes are endlessly versatile. You can chop, stew, broil, bake, or can them, add them to salads, create sauces, and eat them raw.

FRUITS

Apple:

Health benefits: Apples help stimulate all body secretions and their ample minerals and vitamins help to strengthen the blood. Some studies show that an apple a day helps reduce skin disease, arthritis, lung problems, and asthma.

Preparation tips: Try to avoid apples that are sprayed with harmful pesticides. One way to do this is to always wash them very well or peel them. However, there are lots of nutrients in the peel. Apple juice is wonderful, as are apple tea and dried apples, and they are delicious sliced into salads, on sandwiches, or baked for dessert.

Avocado:

Health benefits: Often recommended for malnutrition because the avocado is a good source of many vitamins and minerals. Good for ulcers, constipation, insomnia, and nervousness.

Preparation tips: Good by itself, with a little fresh lemon juice, and in both fruit and vegetable salads. Avacado is the main ingredient in guacamole.

Banana: **Health benefits:** Good for stomach ulcers, colitis, diarrhea, hemorrhoids, and for energy. Some studies show that the inner surface of the skin is beneficial if directly applied to burns or boils.

Preparation tips: Excellent just peeled, but also delicious baked in breads, cakes, and muffins. Do not forget that they are the main component in banana splits and make great-tasting pies and puddings.

Grape: **Health benefits:** Very good internal body cleansers. Excellent for body- and blood-building and as a source of quick energy. Used in some cases of constipation, gout, rheumatism, and skin and liver disorders.

Preparation tips: Most often eaten alone. Make sure you wash them well. You can also toss them into salads, make jams and jellies, and enjoy the sweet flavor of the juice. Grape juice is excellent as a wine substitute in many religious ceremonies.

Orange: **Health benefits:** Recommended for asthma, bronchitis, tuberculosis, pneumonia, rheumatism, arthritis, and high blood pressure. Good for reducing hunger pangs and food cravings. Good for releasing toxins through the skin.

Preparation tips: Best when peeled and eaten in slices or cut into sections, and is also tasty in fruit salad. Orange juice is probably the most common beverage at breakfast, and you may also find the peel candied as a sweet treat.

Pear: **Health benefits:** Used for constipation, poor digestion, high blood pressure, and obesity. Shown to be helpful for skin conditions and colitis, an inflamed condition of the colon.

Preparation tips: Eat pears fresh and remember to wash the skins thoroughly. Pear desserts such as cobblers and brown Betty are very good, as are pear jam, pie, and juice.

GRAINS

Barley: **Health benefits:** Barley is good for gaining weight, helps relieve stomach ulcers, relieves diarrhea, helps prevent tooth decay and hair loss, and improves the condition of finger- and toenails. It is useful in some cases of asthma.

Preparation tips: As a breakfast cereal, use 3 to 4 cups of water to 1 cup barley. For extra flavor, add raisins and milk when done cooking.

Millet: **Health benefits:** Valuable for constipation and for weight gain. Millet is easily digested because it has a low starch content.

Preparation tips: Good for breakfast cereal with nuts, dried fruits, or milk. Use 1 cup millet to 2¼ cups water.

Oats: **Health benefits:** Good for muscle development and as a general body nutritive. Helpful for glands, teeth, hair, and nails.

Oats contain vitamin E, which is good for the heart.

Preparation tips: Oatmeal is a very popular breakfast food and is enhanced when you add raisins, fruit, and milk. Also good in cobblers, cookies, breads, and muffins. Use 1 cup oats to 2 cups water.

Rice: **Health benefits:** Far healthier than its processed white cousin, brown rice is an excellent source of necessary carbohydrates. Brown rice contains many vitamins and minerals and is good for hair, teeth, nails, muscles, and bones.

Preparation tips: Use 1 cup rice to 2 cups water (same for white rice). Rice is the food base of many cultures, including most Asian and African countries. You can make rice into cereal, cakes, cookies, crackers, muffins, waffles, and puddings. Good as a side dish mixed with vegetables or as an accompaniment to stir-fries.

Wheat: **Health benefits:** Wheat is a superb source of the B-complex vitamins. Often recommended in cases of arthritis, rheumatic fever, and even some types of cancer.

Preparation tips: Whole-wheat flour is excellent for baking. Buying the flour is easy, but to ensure that you are getting the most nutrients, buy the grain whole and grind it yourself in a blender or food processor.

NUTS

Almond:

Health benefits: Known to be excellent muscle and body builders. Contains ample amounts of fat, carbohydrate, and protein, and is good for strengthening the body.

Preparation tip: Excellent as butter or milk and as a substitute for sweets and other snack foods. Great in cakes, breads, and salads of vegetables and fruit.

Brazil Nut:

Health benefits: These nuts contain lots of calcium, so they are good for bones and teeth. As with all nuts, they contain lots of fat and are good for treating malnutrition. If you have never tried a Brazil nut before, watch for signs of an allergic reaction as they can be highly allergenic to some people. The signs include hives, a rash, tightening in the chest, and inability to breathe. A shot of epinephrine (adrenaline) helps open the lungs.

Preparation tips: Excellent in baked goods or eaten right out of the shell. Try in baked apples, cookies, muffins, and trail mix.

Cashew Nut:

Health benefits: Good for cases of emaciation, and problems with gums and teeth.

Preparation tips: Roasted cashews are used often in trail mix and baked items. They are best when eaten with acidic fruits and nonstarchy vegetables. Never eat a raw cashew nut, as they are very dangerous.

Filbert: **Health benefits:** These nuts, also known as hazelnuts, form acid in your body and you should eat them in moderation. Good for teeth, gums, and generally strong bodies.

Preparation tips: Filberts are great right out of the shell or in baked goods. The nuts go bad pretty quickly, so leave them in the shell or refrigerate.

Macadamia: **Health benefits:** This nut contains protein, fat, and a enormous amount of calories and carbohydrates. It also has lots of calcium, iron, and phosphorus. Good for anemia and general body strengthening.

Preparation tips: Excellent raw or in baked goods and salads.

Peanut: **Health benefits:** Another high-protein and high-calorie nut, peanuts are great for general nourishment and for treating low blood pressure and low energy.

Preparation tips: Most people have tried peanut butter on a sandwich or a celery stalk, but the nuts are also good in stir-fries, salads, and baked goods, and sprinkled on top of frozen yogurt. Just remember that they are very high in fat and can be very allergenic.

PART FOUR

PUTTING IT ALL TOGETHER: RECIPES AND RESOURCES

— 6 —
WHAT'S COOKIN'?

We want cooking and eating to be fun.

—Mollie Katzen, cookbook author

THE kitchen can be a scary and daunting place if you are not familiar with it. Many teens grow up in families that view cooking as a group activity, where everyone gathers on a Sunday afternoon to chat, taste, and experiment. While your family members may spend quality time preparing meals, they may not be well versed in vegetarian fare. In some homes, where cooking is not something the group does together, one parent may be delegated to the role of family chef. Other families may use the kitchen primarily for heating up frozen foods in the microwave.

Whether you come from a family that cooks or one that is better at making restaurant reservations, learning to create quick and tasty vegetarian dishes can be quite simple. You may be surprised at how fast your family becomes interested in your creations, wondering whether they can share in the delicious fare. Keep in mind, however, that as with any type of cooking, vegetarian foods take some thought and time to prepare.

A common complaint from new vegetarians, young and old, is the lack of variety in vegetarian cooking. In truth, once you begin to peruse vegetarian cookbooks and magazines, you will be amazed at the overwhelming variety and scope of choices. If you think tofu and sprouts are your only options, take a quick glance at the recipes in this chapter and then check out some other cookbooks. You will discover a world of delectable, affordable, and easy-to-prepare snacks, soups, entrées, desserts, and more.

When you begin to cook as a vegetarian, your ideas about entrées, salads, and other foods may change. So might your opinion about what is for lunch and what is for dinner. If you thought soups were just something you ate for lunch or before a meal, you will be surprised to discover that many soups make very satisfying main courses with some bread and salad. What you are striving for when you cook is a healthy meal plan, one that includes a good mix of nutrients from a variety of foods.

The recipes and simple menus in this book were compiled with a busy teen's schedule in mind. While not all foods take less than fifteen minutes to prepare (soups can take a little longer than English muffin pizzas), most do not require you to spend too much time in the kitchen. As you begin to explore vegetarian cooking, you may find that you will want to try more challenging dishes and tastes. There are numerous cookbooks that can guide you toward more complex and elaborate foods. Check the reference section for some of these books or just ask at your local bookstore for more sources.

Most of all, as Mollie Katzen says, cooking and eating should be fun. I hope the sampling of recipes in this chapter will whet your appetite and tickle your curiosity.

GLOSSARY OF COOKING TERMS

BEFORE YOU ENTER the kitchen armed with the vegetarian recipes in this chapter, it will be helpful to know a few cooking terms. Listed here are some key terms you may come across.

al dente: Pasta or vegetables cooked just enough to remain somewhat firm.

blanch: To cook food, usually vegetables, for a few minutes in boiling water. Blanching can also refer to loosening skin so as to remove it, as in blanching almonds.

dice: To cut food into cubes for cooking. Chinese food is often diced for uniform cooking.

dry ingredients: This term generally refers to the "dry" components in recipes, such as flour, baking powder, salt, baking soda, and sugar. Recipes sometimes call for you to combine the dry ingredients before adding milk, butter, or other parts of a batter or mixture.

garnish: Something added to a dish for extra flavor or color; for example, a sprig of parsley on top of mushroom barley soup.

gluten: Used as a meat substitute, gluten is a mixture of plant proteins found primarily in cereal grains from corn and wheat.

purée: Puréeing ingredients, until they have a soupy, liquid consistency, is best achieved by putting the food in a blender or food processor, or rubbing it through a strainer.

saucepan: Usually a deep, straight-sided cooking pot with a handle.

sauté: This cooking technique calls for you to lightly fry ingredients in a shallow pan or a wok, usually with a little bit of fat.

simmer: To gently cook food below the boiling point. Usually you simmer stews and sauces for maximum flavor.

to taste: This term means that you season a dish to your own personal taste. Some people prefer more salt, some like more pepper, and some like a lot of garlic. When a recipe says "season to taste," take a little taste now and then to figure out which seasonings you want to add to enhance flavor.

tofu: Cakes of bean curd made from soybeans.

TVP: Textured vegetable protein. Mix TVP with water and use in place of hamburger. Also good for meatless meatballs, sloppy joes, and vegetarian tacos.

wok: A traditional Asian cooking pan. The bottom can be curved or flat, depending on the type you choose. Woks are excellent for steaming and frying, especially stir-frying. You can also use woks when camping for frying eggs, boiling pasta, and sautéing vegetables.

COOKING TERM ABBREVIATIONS

fl.	fluid
lb.	pound
ml.	milliliter
oz.	ounce
Tbsp.	Tablespoon
tsp.	teaspoon

LIQUID MEASUREMENT CHART

1 cup	8 fl. oz.	½ pint	237.0 ml
2 cups	16 fl. oz.	1 pint	474.0 ml
4 cups	32 fl. oz.	1 quart	946.0 ml
2 pints	32 fl. oz.	1 quart	0.946 liters
4 quarts	128 fl. oz.	1 gallon	3.784 liters

◇ Measure liquids with a standard measuring cup with a spout. For exact measurements, place cup on a level surface and check at eye level.

◇ You can use standard measuring spoons for both liquid and dry measurements.

◇ To accurately measure dry ingredients, use a measuring cup and spoon in the dry ingredient. Do not scoop it. Once the cup is full, level it off with a knife.

Soups

Of soup and love, the first is best.

—Thomas Fuller, seventeenth-century
English writer and clergyman

Soups can take a little more time to prepare than a peanut butter sandwich, but they are a terrific way to make a meal out of fresh, delicious ingredients. You can make a large quantity of soup, freeze it, then reheat it any time you feel like having a bowl. Soups are also endlessly versatile. If you feel like adding something that sounds good to you, like turnips in a vegetable barley soup or pea pods in egg drop soup, go ahead. Like stews, soups often become more tasty the longer they cook and also the next day.

So remember, soup from scratch is not for a situation when you have only 20 minutes to eat, but you can certainly reheat and enjoy a delicious bowl in that time.

LENTIL SOUP

- 1 large onion, chopped
- 2 small carrots, chopped
- 1–2 Tbsp. vegetable oil
- 1½ cups lentils, sorted and washed
- 6 cups vegetable stock* *or* water
  salt, pepper, basil, and parsley, to taste
- 1 large potato, peeled and diced

Sauté onions and carrots in oil until onion is limp. Add lentils, vegetable stock, and seasonings, and bring to a boil.

Cover and lower heat. Simmer for 30 minutes.

Add potato and simmer another 30 minutes, until lentils are very soft.

4–6 servings.

Courtesy of the North American Vegetarian Society

*To make vegetable stock, bring 8 cups water to a boil and add 3 carrots (with skin and greens), 4 stalks celery, 2 large potatoes (with skin), 1 turnip, 4 onions, 4 cloves garlic, 10 mushrooms, 2 Tbsp. olive oil, 1 cup shredded lettuce, 1 tsp. sugar, and salt and pepper to taste. Let mixture simmer for 4 hours and then drain liquid. Discard vegetables or use for Vegetable Barley Soup. Save stock for other soups that would normally require chicken stock.

Egg Drop Soup

2 Tbsp. sesame oil
3 scallions, finely chopped
2 cloves garlic, minced
2 cups vegetable stock *or*
  1 cup stock and 1 cup water
1 tsp. powdered ginger
3 egg whites, beaten*
  salt and pepper, to taste

Heat sesame oil in a frying pan and add chopped scallions and garlic. Sauté until scallions and garlic are just starting to brown. Set aside in a bowl.

Bring vegetable stock to a boil in a medium saucepan. Add powdered ginger. Turn down to a gentle boil. Slowly add beaten egg whites to vegetable stock and watch as they separate into "drops."

Serve soup hot with scallion-and-garlic mixture sprinkled on top.

4 servings.

*To separate eggs, crack egg in half very gently over a bowl. Slowly pour egg from one side of the shell to the other. The white portion will slip into the bowl, while the yolk remains in the shell. Save yolks for omelettes or baking.

VEGETABLE BARLEY SOUP

1 ½ cups water
½ cup barley
5 cups water
3 large carrots, diced
4 stalks celery, diced
2 medium potatoes, unpeeled, diced
10 mushrooms, sliced
1 cup milk (optional)
2 Tbsp. olive oil
3 medium white onions, chopped
4 cloves garlic, minced
½ cup chopped Italian (flat leaf) parsley
½ tsp. oregano
½ tsp. powdered mustard
    salt and pepper, to taste
¼ tsp. chopped chives (for garnish)

Bring 1½ cups water and barley to boil in a covered medium saucepan. Reduce heat and let simmer 30 to 40 minutes.

Place 5 cups of water in a large saucepan. Add carrots, celery, potatoes, and mushrooms. Add barley and milk; bring to a slow boil and stir occasionally.

Sauté onions, garlic, parsley, oregano, mustard, salt, and pepper in olive oil until onions are clear. Add to slow-boiling vegetable-and-barley mixture.

Let soup cook for 30 or 40 minutes. If it is too thick, add more water until you are happy with the consistency. Serve hot with chives on top.

6 servings.

HOT CORN AND POTATO SOUP

4 cups vegetable stock *or* water
3 large carrots, diced with skins
4 stalks celery, diced
1 large onion, chopped
2 medium potatoes, chopped with
   skins
2 Tbsp. butter
2 cups fresh (cooked) *or* frozen
   (defrosted) corn kernels
1 tsp. chili powder
1 tsp. thyme (dried, not fresh)
½ tsp. garlic powder
   salt and pepper, to taste
1 cup milk
   chopped chives, for garnish

Place vegetable stock, carrots, celery, onion, potatoes, and butter in a large pot and bring to a boil. Reduce heat and let simmer.

Add corn, chili powder, thyme, garlic powder, salt, pepper, and milk. Stir well. Let soup simmer for 20 to 30 minutes.

Serve hot with chives on top.

6 servings.

TARRAGON-SCENTED WHITE BEAN SOUP

1 ½ cups dried white beans, picked over
    for rotten beans, and rinsed; soaked
    overnight in ample water to cover
1 Tbsp. safflower *or* canola oil
1 cup thinly sliced leeks *or* coarsely
    chopped onions
6 cups unsalted vegetable stock *or* water
3 medium carrots, halved lengthwise and
    sliced into half moons (semicircles)
2 large ribs celery, diced
2 large bay leaves
2 tsps. dried tarragon leaves
1 tsp. salt, or to taste
    freshly ground pepper, to taste

Drain and rinse the beans. Set aside.

In a heavy 4-quart (or larger) soup pot, heat the oil. Sauté the
leeks for 1 minute, stirring frequently. Add the beans,
water, carrots, celery, bay leaves, and tarragon. Bring to a
boil. Cover and reduce heat to simmer. Cook until the
beans are very tender, about 45 minutes to 1½ hours,
depending upon the size and age of the beans.

Remove the bay leaves. Add salt and pepper to taste. If the
soup is too thin, purée about a cup of the beans and vegetables and return to the soup. If the soup is too thick, add
a little more water or stock. (The soup will thicken con-
siderably upon standing and after refrigeration.)

6 servings.

*Courtesy of Lorna J. Sass, Ph.D.,
and the North American Vegetarian Society*

CREAM OF BROCCOLI SOUP

    2 cups vegetable stock
    1 Tbsp. butter *or* margarine
    1 head broccoli, finely chopped (use
      blender or food processor)
    ½ cup onion, chopped
    1½ cups milk
    1½ Tbsp. cornstarch
    ½ cup milk
      freshly ground pepper, for garnish

Put vegetable stock into medium pot and warm.

Melt butter in a frying pan. Sauté broccoli and onion. Add to
vegetable stock and simmer for 20 minutes. Add 1½ cups
milk and bring to a boil.

In a separate bowl, dissolve cornstarch into ½ cup of milk.
Slowly stir mixture into soup. Continue to boil for 1 or 2
minutes.

Serve with freshly ground pepper on top.

4 servings.

SALADS

'Twas a good lady; we may pick a
thousand salads, ere we light on
such another herb.

—William Shakespeare,
All's Well That Ends Well

MANY VEGETARIANS THINK that from the moment they stop eating meat, life will be one big boring salad—breakfast, lunch, and dinner will consist of an overflowing bowl of not-too-tasty greens. With a little effort and creativity, salads will certainly not be the main ingredient in your diet. Keep in mind though that *salad* is a general term; almost any food you can think of can be included in a salad. Try tossing a few apple and pear slices into your next green salad, as well as raisins and nuts for a little texture.

Salads can be quick, just a few chopped vegetables in a bowl with a dash of oil and vinegar, or they can be complex with roasted garlic, sautéed beans, and baked nuts. They are welcome either before or after a meal, and can even stand as the main course, perhaps accompanied by bread and a bowl of soup. How many times have you opened a menu and seen "Soup and Salad" as an option?

So remember, just because you may begin to eat more salads than you used to, you are not resigned to a life of lettuce. Salads are one area of cooking where an open mind and a vivid imagination are the best ingredients.

TIPS FOR BETTER SALADS

◇After washing greens, place them in the freezer for 10 minutes. It will increase their crunchiness.

◇Make sure you dry lettuce leaves well after washing them or dressing will not cling to them.

◇If you are using cucumbers, soak slices in salted ice water for 30 minutes to make them extra crisp. Do not forget to pat them dry before adding dressing.

◇Greens will keep well in the refrigerator after you have washed them if you wrap them in a paper or cloth towel and place them in a plastic bag.

◇To ensure an even coating of salad dressing, toss your salad in a plastic bag.

◇If you want to keep a portion of a green salad overnight, leave it undressed and store it in the refrigerator.

NOT JUST A GREEN SALAD

1 head lettuce (try romaine, Boston,
    or red leaf lettuce)
2 stalks celery
2 carrots
1 cucumber
5 radishes
2 scallions
1 green, red, *or* yellow bell pepper
1 ripe tomato
1 cup shredded red cabbage
1 cup chickpeas
one 8-oz. can sliced water chestnuts, drained
½ cup sunflower seeds

Dressing:

½ cup olive oil
¼ cup balsamic *or* red wine vinegar
2 Tbsp. water
1 tsp. mustard, prepared
    salt and pepper, to taste
    herbs (oregano, chopped basil,
    rosemary, Italian seasonings)
    chopped fresh garlic *or* garlic powder

Whisk dressing ingredients together in a small bowl *or* measuring cup.

Wash and dry salad greens. Chop all vegetables and toss with greens in a large bowl. Add chickpeas and water chestnuts.

Dress salad 15 minutes before serving. Sprinkle with sunflower seeds.

4–6 servings.

Cold Pasta Salad

> 4 cups cooked pasta—use a short
>   pasta (e.g., penne, rigatoni, far-
>   falle) *not* spaghetti or lasagna
> 1 onion, chopped fine
> 2 cups fresh vegetables (carrots, cel-
>   ery, zucchini, cabbage, green or
>   red bell pepper, mushrooms, etc.)
> 1 cup cooked beans (kidney, gar-
>   banzo, lentils, etc.)
>
> **Dressing:**
> ½ cup vegetable oil
> ½ cup vinegar
>   salt, pepper, and other seasonings,
>   to taste

Combine pasta with onion, vegetables, and beans.

Mix dressing ingredients together and pour over pasta mixture. Toss well. Chill before serving.

4-6 servings

Courtesy of the North American Vegetarian Society

TOMATO AND ONION SALAD WITH FETA CHEESE

    6 large tomatoes
    ½ large red onion
    ½ lb. feta cheese
    1 cup fresh basil leaves, chopped
       salt and pepper, to taste

Chop tomatoes and onion. Toss in medium bowl.

Sprinkle feta cheese and basil on tomato-and-onion mixture.

Toss and season with salt and pepper.

4 servings.

Courtesy of Jane S. Ferber

BOUNTIFUL BEAN SALAD

3 cups cooked *or* canned beans, such
   as black turtles, rattlesnakes, *or* pintos
½ cup diced red bell pepper
⅓ cup finely chopped onion *or* scallions
½ cup pimento-stuffed olives,
   coarsely chopped
¼ cup tightly packed minced fresh
   coriander *or* parsley
4–5 Tbsp. lime juice, divided
   salt, to taste
2 Tbsp. olive oil
   radicchio leaves arranged as cups,
   for garnish
   avocado slices, for garnish

In a bowl, combine the beans, bell pepper, onion, olives,
coriander, 3 Tbsp. lime juice, and salt to taste. Allow to
sit at room temperature for 1 to 2 hours.

Just before serving, stir in olive oil and enough additional
lime juice to give the salad a sharp edge.

Mound salad into radicchio cups and garnish with avocado
slices.

Note: After overnight refrigeration, this salad will need to be
perked up with an additional tablespoon or two of fresh
lime juice. Serve at room temperature.

4 servings.

*Courtesy of Lorna J. Sass, Ph.D., and the North American
Vegetarian Society*

"PICK-ME-UP" POTATO SALAD

6 medium potatoes
4 scallions, chopped
3 stalks celery, chopped
¼ cup chopped green bell pepper
¼ cup chopped red bell pepper
¼ cup chopped black olives
2 Tbsp. finely chopped parsley
2 cups plain yogurt
 salt, pepper, and garlic powder to
 taste

Boil potatoes until soft and chop into medium-sized pieces. Allow to cool to room temperature.

Add all other ingredients to the potatoes. Add salt, pepper, and garlic according to taste.

6–8 servings.

Main Dishes

It's food too fine for angels; yet come,
take
And eat thy fill!

—Edward Taylor, Colonial American poet
and author of "Poetical Works"

THE LIST OF vegetarian and vegan entrées grows larger each year. As more professional and lay chefs devote their energies to meatless and dairyless recipes, the variety of main dishes increases. You can definitely make a wholesome and hearty meal of soup, salad, and bread, but it is also fun to cook something a little different and adventurous once in a while. As you begin to experiment with more flavors and ingredients, you will become better at mixing and matching to satisfy your own tastes. Recipes are good starting points when learning to cook. After you feel confident, there is no end to what you can create in the kitchen.

Whipping up a meal is often more fun with company. If you decide to make vegetable lasagna or vegetarian chili, ask a member of your family to help out or a friend to keep you company. While some people enjoy the solitary experience of cooking, most like to chat and have tasters around.

The best place to start with these, as with any recipe, is with the freshest ingredients you can find. If you cannot locate a health food store near you, remember that your local supermarket may have fresh and even organic produce and grains. Several chains across the country, such as Key Food in New York and Fresh Fields in Pennsylvania, are beginning to carry a growing selection of organic products.

Vegetable Lasagna

one 1-lb. package lasagna noodles,
    cooked and drained
  2 eggplants, peeled and sliced into
    thin rounds
  2 tomatoes, sliced
  1 green zucchini, sliced into thin
    rounds
  1 yellow squash, sliced into thin rounds
  1 cup minced onion
 ½ cup minced garlic
 ½ cup minced parsley
 ½ cup minced basil
two 14-oz. jars of your favorite tomato
    sauce
one 10-oz. box semisoft tofu, sliced

Preheat oven to 350°F.

Combine all vegetable ingredients and seasoning in one bowl. Cover the bottom of a 9" × 13" lasagna pan with a thin layer of tomato sauce. Add a layer of lasagna noodles. Top with an even layer of vegetables. Cover lightly with another layer of tomato sauce. Continue layering noodles and vegetables, always covering the vegetables with some sauce, until they have all been used. Top with tofu slices and remaining tomato sauce.

Bake for 1 hour.

8–10 servings.

Courtesy of Lena and Marc Romanoff

EMPEROR'S EGGPLANT

- ¼ cup sesame oil
- ½ cup soy sauce
- 6 cloves garlic, chopped
- ½ cup each green, yellow, and red bell pepper, chopped
- ½ cup parsley, chopped
- 4 Tbsp. chives
- 4 baby eggplants
    sesame seeds, for garnish
- 10 cherry tomatoes, for garnish

Mix sesame oil, soy sauce, garlic, bell peppers, parsley, and chives in a bowl, cover, and refrigerate for 6 hours.

Steam baby eggplants until tender. Cool and split in half, keeping the skin on.

Pour reserved mixture on top of eggplant. Arrange on a platter. Sprinkle with sesame seeds. Garnish with cherry tomatoes.

4 servings.

Courtesy of Lena and Marc Romanoff

Party "Meatball" Skewers

1 box Boca Vegan Burgers
2 Tbsp. olive oil
½ cup bread crumbs *or* matzoh meal
2 cups cubed fresh *or* canned pineapple
one 8-oz. can whole water chestnuts
6 bamboo skewers

Preheat oven to 250°F.

Make several small "meatballs" from Boca burgers. Dip each "meatball" in bread crumbs.

Gently sauté the meatballs in the olive oil for 5 to 10 minutes. Set aside to cool.

When cooled, alternate meatballs, pineapple, and water chestnuts on skewers. Place on baking sheet lined with aluminum foil. Heat in oven for 10 minutes.

Serve with Mango Sauce or ketchup.

Mango Sauce:

2 ripe mangos, mashed
⅓ cup soy sauce
4 Tbsp. currant jelly
3 tsp. lemon juice
½ cup plain yogurt

Blend ingredients together and serve as a dipping sauce.

4 servings.

Courtesy of Lena and Marc Romanoff

Vegetarian Chili

        4 tsps. olive oil
    1 ½ cups chopped onion
        4 cloves garlic, minced
        5 tsp. chili powder
    1 ¾ tsp. ground cumin
        ½ tsp. salt
        ½ tsp. freshly ground pepper
        ½ tsp. dried oregano
⅛–¼ tsp. red pepper flakes
        ⅛ tsp. ground red pepper
        2 cups each large red and green bell
            pepper cubes
        1 cup cubed carrot
        ¼ cup water
        4 cups drained canned tomatoes,
            coarsely chopped
        1 cup tomato purée *or* canned
            tomatoes, drained and puréed in a
            blender or food processor
        2 cups cubed zucchini
            one 14-oz. can pinto *or* red kidney
            beans, drained

In a large pot, heat oil over medium heat. Add onion and gar-
    lic. Sauté until tender. Stir in seasonings and herbs. Cook
    30 seconds.

Stir in bell peppers, carrot, and water; cover and cook 10
    minutes or until tender. Add chopped tomatoes and
    tomato purée.

Bring to a boil, cover, reduce heat to low, and simmer 30 minutes. Stir in zucchini and beans. Cover and cook 5 minutes.

4 servings.

Courtesy of Carol Jacobanis

GREEN FETTUCCINE WITH GOAT CHEESE, BROCCOLI, AND CAULIFLOWER

    2 cups broccoli florets (just the tops,
      not the stems)
    2 cups cauliflower florets (just the
      tops, not the stems)
 1 ½ cups vegetable stock
    8 oz. goat cheese
    2 tsp. fresh, chopped thyme
    ½ tsp. salt
    ¼ tsp. white pepper
    1 Tbsp. oil
    ¾ pound spinach fettuccine, fresh
    1 Tbsp. finely chopped, fresh parsley,
      for garnish

Immerse broccoli and cauliflower in a large pan of boiling water and boil about 5 minutes or until cooked but slightly crunchy. Drain and pour cold water over vegetables to stop the cooking process. Drain thoroughly. In a 9-inch skillet, boil vegetable stock until reduced to 1 cup, about 15 minutes.

Scrape rind off cheese with a knife, removing as thin a layer as possible. Cut cheese into small pieces. Whisk goat cheese into stock. Add thyme, salt, and pepper. Simmer about 5 minutes until slightly thickened. Taste for seasoning. Add broccoli and cauliflower, reserving 6 florets of each.

Add oil to a large pot of boiling water. Add pasta and cook
until al dente, about 30 seconds. Drain well. Place in skillet of sauce and toss until well combined.

Put in serving bowl or on plates and garnish with reserved
florets and parsley.

2–3 servings.

Courtesy of Carol Jacobanis

Potato Pie

3 medium potatoes, peeled and cut
    into chunks
¼ cup water
½ tsp. salt
⅛ tsp. black pepper
1 tsp. vegetable oil
1 Tbsp. vegetable oil
1 onion, diced
1 head broccoli, cut into florets
1 green bell pepper, diced
4 medium carrots, diced
1 cup frozen peas
1 cup chopped fresh tomatoes
½ tsp. basil
1 tsp. salt
2 cups collard greens *or* kale,
    chopped
½ tsp. paprika

Preheat oven to 350°F.

Steam or boil potatoes until soft. Mash, adding water, salt, pepper, and 1 tsp. oil. Set aside.

Sauté onion in 1 Tbsp. oil for a few minutes. Add broccoli, bell pepper, carrots, peas, tomatoes, basil, and salt. Bring to a boil; cover and simmer until vegetables are tender, about 15 minutes. Add greens and cook for another 5 minutes.

Put vegetables into a medium baking dish. Top with mashed
potatoes and sprinkle with paprika.

Bake for 10 to 15 minutes and serve.

6 servings.

Courtesy of the North American Vegetarian Society

STIR-FRIES

Stir-frying is one of the best ways to create delicious, healthy meals in the shortest possible time.

—Joie Warner, cookbook author

YOU CAN MAKE stir-fries, like salads, out of almost anything you can think up. The key is to get the freshest ingredients possible; use a Chinese cooking pan, or wok; and be ready to eat your creation almost immediately. Most recipes for stir-fries derive from Chinese cooking, but you can prepare other dishes with the same method of cooking at high heat for a brief period of time.

Not every stir-fry will taste exactly as you expect, but it is good to keep experimenting with new ingredients and different techniques. Some points to keep in mind include: cook small pieces very quickly over very high heat, so that vegetables do not lose their flavor or nutritional value through excessive heat; always use a wok (if you do not have access to a wok, use a large nonstick skillet); and cut vegetables and tofu, if you use it, into uniform shapes so they will all finish cooking around the same time. It is also a good idea to have everything you plan on using chopped and ready to go into the wok before you begin heating any oil.

Most major cities and suburbs have Asian markets where you can buy unusual ingredients that you have never tried before for your stir-fries. Some new foods you may encounter include bamboo shoots, bean curd or tofu, sesame oil, black bean sauce, and straw mushrooms. If you are limited to ingredients at your supermarket, remember to look for the ones that look freshest. Stir-fries are a lot of fun to make and it is easy for you to get a lot of different nutrients from one tasty dish.

BROCCOLI AND TOFU STIR-FRY
WITH BLACK BEAN SAUCE

- 1 head broccoli
- 4 cakes tofu (try to get fresh, but if unavailable use packaged)
- 1 Tbsp. vegetable oil
- 3 cloves garlic, minced
- 1 onion, chopped
- 3 scallions, chopped
  salt and pepper to taste
- 2 Tbsp. black bean sauce

Chop broccoli florets and stalks into medium-size pieces. Cut tofu into medium-size cubes. Set aside.

Heat oil in a wok over medium to high heat; sauté garlic, onion, scallions, salt, and pepper until the onion is clear and the garlic just turning brown. Add tofu. Let tofu become crispy on all sides.

Add broccoli and cook over high heat for a few minutes, until broccoli is bright green.

Turn down heat and add black bean sauce. Cover and cook over low heat for 2 minutes. Serve immediately with brown rice.

4 servings.

Stir-Fried Asparagus with Yellow and Red Pepper in Sesame Oil

1 ample bunch of asparagus
  (10–12 spears)
1 yellow bell pepper
1 red bell pepper
2 Tbsp. sesame oil
2 cloves garlic, minced
1 medium onion, chopped
½ teaspoon powdered ginger
2 Tbsp. soy sauce
one 8-oz. can bamboo shoots, drained
1 scallion, chopped, for garnish

Cut asparagus into 1-inch pieces, discarding bottom ends. Cut peppers into 1-inch slivers, discarding all seeds.

Heat oil in wok over high heat. Cook garlic, onion, and ginger for about 2 minutes.

Add asparagus and peppers. Cook over high heat for 1 minute. Add soy sauce and toss mixture. Add bamboo shoots and reduce heat. Cover and cook for another minute or two.

Sprinkle with scallion. Serve immediately with brown rice.

2 servings.

GREEN BEANS, TOFU, AND PEANUTS WITH SPICY SAUCE

1 lb. green beans
4 cakes tofu
2 Tbsp. vegetable oil
3 cloves garlic, minced
½ tsp. powdered ginger
salt and pepper, to taste
1 Tbsp. chili paste
1 cup unsalted peanuts

Remove ends of green beans. Cut tofu into ½-inch cubes. Set aside.

Heat oil in wok over high heat. Add garlic, ginger, salt, and pepper. Cook for 30 seconds. Add beans, tofu, and chili paste. Cook for 1 minute and add peanuts. Toss and cook for another 30 seconds.

Serve immediately with brown rice.

4 servings.

"PEAS PLEASE" STIR-FRY

1 lb. fresh snow peas
2 cups frozen green peas
1 red bell pepper, diced
1 Tbsp. vegetable oil
2 cloves garlic, minced
1 Tbsp. fresh ginger, finely chopped
salt and pepper, to taste
one 8-oz. can sliced water chestnuts,
    drained
soy sauce

Remove ends from fresh snow peas. Cook frozen peas in boiling water. Set aside.

Heat oil in wok over high flame. Add garlic, ginger, salt, and pepper. Cook for a few seconds.

Add peas and bell pepper and cook on high heat for 1 minute. Reduce heat and add water chestnuts. Cover and cook for 30 seconds more.

Add splash of soy sauce. Serve immediately with brown rice.

4 servings.

CHINESE EGGPLANT WITH KIDNEY BEANS AND OYSTER SAUCE

3 Chinese *or* regular eggplants
1 green bell pepper
3 Tbsp. vegetable oil
2 cloves garlic, minced
½ tsp. powdered ginger
1 large onion, chopped
one 15-oz. can red kidney beans, drained
2 Tbsp. oyster sauce

Cut ends off eggplants. Cut remaining chunks into 2-inch pieces. Cut bell pepper into slivers. Set aside.

Heat oil in wok over high heat. Cook garlic, ginger, and onion until onion is clear and garlic is crispy.

Add eggplant and cook for about 4 minutes. Add bell pepper and cook another minute. Add kidney beans and toss. Reduce heat and cook another 30 seconds.

Add oyster sauce, stir, and serve immediately with brown rice.

4 servings.

SIDE DISHES

What I say is that, if a man really likes potatoes, he must be a pretty decent sort of fellow.

—A. A. Milne
Not That It Matters

MANY PEOPLE THINK that potatoes are the only side dishes out there. Potatoes make excellent sides to many of the meals you create, but they are certainly not the only ones. In fact, not all main courses will need a side dish, but sometimes you may just want to make one anyway. Sides are not snacks per se, but if you have a few minutes and want to eat something that is not too filling, try whipping up one of the following recipes for a quick treat.

When you cook side dishes, you usually do not make an enormous quantity because they are supposed to complement another, more substantial dish. Many vegetarians discover, when they attend a dinner party or another function where there are no vegetarian options, that side dishes make a pretty good meal on their own. Most are either vegetable- or starch-based and the variety is endless.

Side dishes make great leftovers, especially when you are pressed for time. Open the fridge, peek inside, and see if anything jumps out at you.

COOKING BEANS AND RICE

A LOT OF the side dishes you cook will have beans and rice in the recipe. Here is an easy-to-follow chart on how to prepare most grains and beans.

Grain/bean (1 dry cup)	Water (in cups)	Cooking Time* (in minutes)	Yield (in cups)
Barley (whole)	3	75	3½
Brown rice	2	40–60	3
Buckwheat	2	15	2½
Cornmeal	4	25	3
White rice	2	30	2
Black beans	4	90	2
Black-eyed peas	3	60	2
Chickpeas	4	180	2
Great Northern beans	3½	120	2
Kidney beans	3	90	2
Lentils/split peas†	3	60	2¼
Lima beans	2	90	1¼
Pinto beans	3	150	2
Red beans	3	180	2

*Cooking times may vary, depending upon the age of the grains or beans.
† Lentils and split peas should not be soaked before cooking.

◇ Soaking beans in water overnight will reduce cooking time.

◇ Beans will be more tender if you add a drop of vinegar or lemon juice to the cooking water.

◇ To turn a pot of beans into stew, add chopped vegetables and herbs for the last half-hour of cooking.

◇ For an easy meal, combine cooked grains and beans with herbs and steamed, stir-fried, or raw vegetables.

◇Try serving beans on a bed of lettuce and rice. Garnish with tomato, carrots, scallions, and the like

Courtesy of the North American Vegetarian Society

Spanish Rice

1 medium onion, chopped
½ cup chopped green bell pepper
2–3 cloves garlic, minced
2–4 Tbsp. vegetable oil
1 cup canned crushed tomatoes
1 tsp. chili powder
1 cup uncooked brown *or* white rice
2 cups water
 salt, pepper, and other seasonings,
 to taste

In a heavy saucepan, sauté onion, pepper, and garlic in oil until onion is transparent. Add tomatoes, chili powder, rice, water, and seasonings.

Bring to a boil, then reduce heat and simmer over very low heat for 30 minutes for brown rice or 20 minutes for white rice. Turn off heat and let sit for 10 minutes. Eat hot or cold.

4 servings.

Courtesy of the North American Vegetarian Society

CORN-RICE PILAF

   3 Tbsp. raisins
  ½ cup boiling water
   1 cup diced celery
   1 onion, chopped
2–4 Tbsp. vegetable oil
  ½ tsp. salt
   1 cup canned corn, drained *or*
      frozen corn, cooked and drained
   4 cups cooked rice

Soak raisins in boiling water to plump them. Set aside.

In a deep skillet, sauté the celery and onion in oil for 5 minutes; add salt and drained raisins. Cook for 2 minutes.

Add corn and rice and heat through. Toss lightly with a fork.

4 servings.

Courtesy of the North American Vegetarian Society

MEXICAN-STYLE LENTILS

1 cup uncooked lentils
2 cups water
1 cup tomato sauce
1 onion, chopped
1 cup canned corn, drained
  salt, pepper, and seasonings, to
  taste

Boil lentils in water for 30 minutes. Drain off extra liquid. Combine all ingredients.

Simmer over low heat for 30 minutes or until lentils are tender. Serve over pasta or rice.

4 servings.

Courtesy of the North American Vegetarian Society

Oven-Roasted Potatoes

 2½ lbs. small red or white rose
     potatoes *or* yellow Finnish potatoes
 ¼ cup vegetable oil
 2 tsp. salt
 ¼ tsp. paprika
 ½ tsp. finely ground pepper

Preheat oven to 425°F.

Peel potatoes, rinse, and pat dry. Cut each potato into eighths or 2-inch wedges.

Combine oil, salt, paprika, and pepper in a bowl and mix well. Add potatoes and toss.

Arrange on an oiled baking sheet and bake 45 minutes, turning every 15 minutes, until tender and well browned. Season to taste. Serve immediately.

(If you want, add chopped fresh herbs, such as rosemary, thyme, or oregano, to the oil mixture. Olive oil may be substituted for vegetable oil. You may also roast the potatoes unpeeled.)

6 servings.

Courtesy of Carol Jacobanis

SAUTÉED CHERRY TOMATOES

2 pints cherry tomatoes, rinsed and
   stemmed
1 ½ Tbsp. sweet butter
½ cup chopped fresh parsley
   salt and pepper, to taste

To make peeling easier, blanch tomatoes in boiling water for
about 1 minute. Remove and rinse under cool water;
skins should slip off easily.

Melt butter (adding a drop of oil, if desired, to prevent burn-
ing) in a large skillet over medium-high heat.

Add tomatoes and sauté *briefly*. Sprinkle with parsley, season to taste with salt and pepper, and serve.

4 servings.

Courtesy of Carol Jacobanis

CHEESE TORTELLINI WITH RED PEPPERS AND ROSEMARY

    2 Tbsp. olive oil
    2 red bell peppers, chopped
    1 medium onion, chopped
      a few sprigs of fresh rosemary
    2 cloves garlic, chopped
      salt and pepper, to taste
    1 lb. fresh cheese tortellini

In a large skillet, heat oil and sauté bell peppers, onion, rosemary, garlic, salt, and pepper. Cook for about 4 minutes and remove from heat.

Bring a large pot of water to boil. Add tortellini. Cook for 2 minutes or until pasta floats to the top.

Drain pasta and transfer to a medium bowl. Add bell pepper mixture and toss. Season to taste.

4 servings.

BREADS

No smell is more welcoming than that of freshly baked bread.

—Julee Rosso and Sheila Lukins, cookbook authors

YOU HAVE PROBABLY been eating bread almost your entire life. Your first sandwich may have been peanut butter and jelly or tuna fish wrapped in wax paper and lovingly placed in your lunch bag. Almost every culture in the world has its own form of bread. In Mexico it is the tortilla, in India the chappati, and in France the baguette. In the United States, many people bake bread on a regular basis, freezing several loaves at a time.

The variety of ingredients that you can include in a loaf made of white or wheat flour is endless. Some people like cheese and herbs, while others may include nuts and bananas. The basics of baking bread are very simple and inexpensive. Bread takes a little while to make because you must allow time for the dough to rise. When you make bread, do it in bulk so you can bake a number of loaves at once. While bread always tastes best fresh, it is also delicious after defrosting.

Basic Whole-Wheat Bread

one ¼-oz. package (2½ tsp.) active dry
    yeast
 ½ tsp. sugar
    small bowl of warm water
 4 cups whole-wheat flour
 2 Tbsp. gluten
 2 tsp. salt
1½ cups rice milk *or* soy milk
 2 Tbsp. molasses
 1 Tbsp. maple syrup
    cornmeal

Preheat oven to 375°F.

Add yeast and sugar to the bowl of warm water. Let sit for about 5 minutes or until mixture is foamy.

Combine flour, gluten, and salt in a big mixing bowl. Pour yeast into flour mixture and mix with a wooden spoon or your hands. When well blended, add milk, molasses, and syrup. Mix well.

Place dough in an oiled bowl and cover with plastic wrap. Let dough rise in a warm spot for 1½ hours or until dough has doubled. After rising, punch dough down and let rise for another hour.

Make loaf out of dough. Sprinkle cornmeal into a 5" × 9" ungreased loaf pan. Place dough in pan and bake for 50 minutes or until a knife inserted in the center of the loaf comes out clean.

Adapted from a recipe by Jennie O. Collura
Courtesy of the North American Vegetarian Society

ROSEMARY FOCACCIA

one ¼-oz. package (2½ tsp.) active dry
   yeast
½ tsp. sugar
1 cup lukewarm water
3½ cups flour
1 tsp. salt
5 Tbsp. olive oil, divided
½ tsp. minced garlic
1 Tbsp. finely chopped fresh rosemary
   leaves, or to taste (plus sprigs for
   garnish)
1 Tbsp. coarse salt

Combine yeast, sugar, and water in a large bowl. Let sit for
about 5 minutes or until mixture is foamy; add flour, salt,
and 3 Tbsp. of the oil and mix well. Knead (by hand or
with dough hook of electric mixer) until soft and slightly
sticky.

Form dough into a ball, transfer to an oiled bowl, and turn it
to coat it with oil. Let rise, covered with plastic wrap or
a cloth sprinkled with flour, in a warm place for 1½ hours
or until doubled in bulk.

Note: The dough may be made up to this point, punched
down, covered, and chilled overnight. Let dough return to
room temperature before proceeding.

Press dough into an oiled 10" × 15" jelly-roll pan. Let rise,
covered loosely, in a warm place for 1 hour or until
almost doubled in bulk.

Preheat oven to 400°F.

In a small bowl stir together the remaining 2 Tbsp. oil, garlic, and rosemary. Dimple the dough, making $\frac{1}{4}$-inch-deep indentations with your fingertips. Brush with the oil mixture and sprinkle with coarse salt. Bake the focaccia in the bottom third of the oven for 35 to 45 minutes or until golden brown. Let cool in pan on rack and garnish with rosemary sprigs. Serve warm or at room temperature.

Courtesy of Carol Jacobanis

CORNBREAD

1 cup flour
1 cup yellow cornmeal
¼ cup sugar
1 Tbsp. baking powder
½ tsp. baking soda
½ tsp. salt
2 eggs, beaten
1 cup buttermilk
¼ cup oil

Preheat oven to 425°F.

Combine dry ingredients. In a separate bowl, combine liquid ingredients.

Add liquid to dry ingredients, stirring just to blend (do not overmix). Pour into 8" × 8" pan greased with oil and bake for 20 minutes.

Cool slightly. May be served warm or at room temperature.

Courtesy of Carol Jacobanis

BLUEBERRY MUFFINS

- 1 egg
- ½ cup milk
- ¼ cup vegetable oil
- 1½ cups flour
- ½ cup sugar
- 2 tsp. baking powder
- ½ tsp. salt
- 1 cup fresh *or* frozen blueberries
  sugar—a few pinches to cover
  muffins

Preheat oven to 400°F.

Slightly beat egg in a bowl. Stir in milk and oil.

Mix flour, sugar, baking powder, and salt together. Stir in just enough of egg mixture to moisten dry ingredients. Batter should be lumpy at this point.

Stir in blueberries.

Fill greased or paper-lined muffin cups ⅔ full. Sprinkle tops with sugar.

Bake for 20 to 25 minutes.

12 muffins.

Courtesy of Carol Jacobanis

DATE–NUT BREAD

1½ cups boiling water
1½ cups dates, cut up
½ cup brown sugar, packed
1 Tbsp. softened butter *or* margarine
1 egg
2¼ cups flour
1 tsp. baking soda
½ tsp. salt
1 cup broken nuts

Preheat oven to 350°F.

Pour water over dates and let cool.

Mix together sugar, butter, and egg. Stir in dates and water.

Sift together flour, baking soda, and salt. Stir into date mixture. Blend in nuts.

Pour mixture into a greased 5" × 9" loaf pan. Let stand 20 minutes. Bake for 60 to 70 minutes.

Courtesy of Carol Jacobanis

SPICED CARROT BREAD

4 eggs
2 cups sugar
1 ¼ cups vegetable oil
3 cups flour
2 tsp. baking powder
1 ½ tsp. baking soda
¼ tsp. salt
2 tsp. cinnamon
¼ tsp. nutmeg
2 cups finely shredded raw carrots
1 cup walnuts

Preheat oven to 350°F.

Grease a 5" × 9" loaf pan. Set aside.

Beat eggs with electric or hand mixer. Gradually add sugar. Add oil. Continue beating until well blended.

Stir in flour, baking powder, baking soda, salt, cinnamon, and nutmeg. Beat until smooth. Stir in carrots and nuts.

Spoon batter into pan, filling no more than ⅔ full. Bake for 50 minutes or until a knife inserted in center of bread comes out clean. Leave bread in pan; cool 10 minutes on a wire rack. Then remove from pan and allow to cool completely.

Courtesy of Carol Jacobanis

DESSERTS

Promises and Pie-Crust
are made to be broken.

—Jonathan Swift,
author of *Gulliver's Travels*

MOST OF THE time it is tempting to skip the main part of a meal and head straight for the dessert tray. There is no doubt a general perception that desserts are bad for people, and that is part of what makes them so appealing to young and old alike. Few desserts have meat in them, so most vegetarians can often enjoy without worry. Vegans may have to check ingredients and ask what is in a type of cake or cookie. It is hard to avoid using dairy products when baking, but it is certainly possible. Besides, baked goods are not the only type of after-dinner treat.

When you concoct a dessert, do not be disappointed if your cake or pie does not look exactly like the one at your local bakery. Baking is not something you pick up immediately, but a skill that you hone as time goes by. A lot of cooking is a little of this and a little of that, but with baked goods, you generally need to measure ingredients precisely. Think of it as chemistry, with all the different elements working together to make a whole. Do not have such high expectations at first and you will not be disappointed with a few fallen cakes or burnt cookies.

If you enlist family members and friends to taste your creations, ask them to be honest about what they are tasting. Their comments will help you improve your technique the next time around.

Apple Oat Crisp

6 apples, peeled, cored, and thinly
   sliced
½ tsp. cinnamon
½ cup brown sugar
1 cup rolled oats
½ cup vegetable oil

Preheat oven to 300°F.

Place apple slices in a lightly oiled 10" casserole dish. Sprinkle with cinnamon and 2 Tbsp. of the sugar.

Combine oats and remaining sugar in a bowl. Add oil and mix the dough with a fork until it is crumbly. Sprinkle over apples.

Bake for 40 minutes, or until topping is brown.

4-6 servings.

Courtesy of the North American Vegetarian Society

CINNAMON RICE DESSERT

1 cup raisins
1 cup boiling water
2 apples
½ cup sugar
½ cup cold water
1 tsp. cinnamon
½ tsp. vanilla
2–3 cups cooked, cooled brown rice
(1½ cups dry)

Soak raisins in boiling water. Set aside.

Core and peel apples and cut into medium-size wedges. In a saucepan, mix sugar and cold water. Add apple slices and cook over medium heat until apples are soft but not mushy. Add cinnamon and vanilla.

Drain raisins and add apple mixture and cooled rice. Stir. Serve warm or chilled.

4 servings.

Courtesy of the North American Vegetarian Society

Baked Apples

6 large baking apples (such as Rome
   or Cortland)
6 tsp. honey
1 cup crushed walnuts
1½ tsp. cinnamon
   vanilla frozen yogurt (optional)

Preheat oven to 300°F.

Scoop out centers of apples, so that you have made a small
bowl in the middle of each apple.

Spoon 1 tsp. honey into each apple; add about 2½ Tbsp.
crushed walnuts and sprinkle with ¼ tsp. cinnamon.

Bake for 15 to 20 minutes or until you can smell the apples.
Serve hot with or without frozen yogurt.

6 servings.

STRAWBERRY SHORTCAKE

Baking Powder Biscuits

2 cups flour
3 tsp. baking powder
1 tsp. salt
¼ cup vegetable shortening
¾ cup milk

Preheat oven to 450°F.

Sift together flour, baking powder, and salt. Cut in shortening until consistency is of coarse meal. Stir milk in lightly, just until blended. Turn dough out onto a floured board and knead gently for a scant 30 seconds.

Pat dough out to ½-inch thick and cut into 6 circles with an upturned glass. Place on a greased baking sheet and bake for 10 to 12 minutes.

Strawberry Topping:

3 pints strawberries
extra-fine sugar, if needed

Wash berries, remove stems, and slice. Set 1 pint sliced berries aside. Mash the remainder with a fork. Add sugar, if needed, to sweeten. Stir in reserved berries.

Chantilly

1 cup whipping cream
½ tsp. vanilla
   powdered sugar (optional)

Whip cream until slightly thickened. Add vanilla and sugar
   as desired and continue whipping to *very* soft peaks.

Assembly:

Split biscuits. Top each biscuit half with strawberries and a
   dollop of whipped cream. Add more or less cream and
   berries as desired.

12 servings.

Courtesy of Carol Jacobanis

CARROT CAKE

1 cup corn oil
2 cups sugar
3 eggs
1 ½ cups shredded carrots
2 cups flour
one 8-oz. can crushed pineapple, drained
1 tsp. baking soda
1 tsp. salt
1 tsp. vanilla
1 tsp. allspice
1 tsp. cinnamon
1 cup chopped walnuts

Preheat oven to 350°F.

Combine all ingredients and blend well. Pour into a 9" × 13" pan lined with waxed paper and bake for 1 hour. Let cool and frost with Cream Cheese Frosting.

Cream Cheese Frosting:

3 oz. butter *or* margarine
3 oz. cream cheese
1 cup powdered sugar
½ tsp. vanilla
1 tsp. lemon juice

Beat all ingredients until fluffy. Spread on cake.

Courtesy of Carol Jacobanis

SNICKERDOODLES

  1 cup soft vegetable shortening
1½ cups sugar
  2 eggs
2¾ cups sifted flour
  2 tsp. cream of tartar
  1 tsp. baking soda
  ¼ tsp. salt
  2 Tbsp. sugar
  2 tsp. cinnamon

Preheat oven to 400°F.

Mix shortening, sugar, and eggs together thoroughly. In a separate bowl, sift together flour, cream of tartar, baking soda, and salt. Stir the two mixtures together to make a dough

Roll dough into balls the size of small walnuts. Roll the balls in a mixture of sugar and cinnamon. Place balls 2 inches apart on an ungreased baking sheet.

Bake about 8 to 10 minutes until lightly brown, but still soft.

Yield depends on size of each snickerdoodle.

Courtesy of Carol Jacobanis

SURPRISE MERINGUES (A.K.A. "POLKA-DOT KISSES")

2 egg whites, at room temperature
⅛ tsp. salt
⅛ tsp. cream of tartar
1 tsp. vanilla
¾ cup sugar
  one 6-oz. package semisweet
  chocolate chips
¼ cup chopped walnuts

Preheat oven to 300°F.

Beat egg whites, salt, cream of tartar, and vanilla until soft peaks form.

Gradually add sugar to egg mixture while beating constantly, until peaks are stiff.

Carefully fold in chocolate chips and walnuts.

Cover a baking sheet with foil. Drop rounded teaspoons of the mixture onto sheet. Bake for about 25 minutes.

Yield will vary.

Courtesy of Carol Jacobanis

BROWN BETTY

Topping

1 cup rolled oats
1 cup whole-wheat flour
¼ cup canola oil
¼ cup maple syrup
¼ cup apple juice
1 tsp. cinnamon

Mix all ingredients together in a bowl. You can make this one day ahead and keep it in the refrigerator.

Filling:

4 cups of fruit, 3 types: apples, pears, bananas, berries, or any combination of these (peel and slice apples, pears, and bananas)
1 cup apple juice, pear juice, or berry juice
1 Tbsp. arrowroot

Preheat oven to 365°F.

Place fruit in a 12" × 12" baking dish. Toss with juice and arrowroot.

Sprinkle topping over the fruit. Bake about 30 minutes, until the filling is tender and bubbling. Top should be golden brown.

6 servings.

Courtesy of Chef Jeanette Maier

SNACKS

Variety's the very spice of life

—William Cowper, eighteenth-century
English poet

IT IS NOT always easy to get in three balanced meals a day, but there seems to be no problem finding time to snack. Most parents assume that their teens snack on junk. You can dispel this misconception by making an effort to create healthy and wholesome snacks that are always on hand to give you an energy boost.

The benefits of making your own snacks include the following: you know exactly what goes into them; you can create them in bulk so they last a while; you can make them with as much variety as you want; and they give you an opportunity to try new combinations of foods. Do not limit yourself to what is lying around in the pantry. Go to your local health food store or ethnic food store and try something new. If you run out of ideas, throw a party where each person has to come with a different snack and its recipe. Gather all the recipes together, copy them, and distribute them to your friends.

Snacks should not be replacements for meals, but for busy teenagers, healthy alternatives to potato chips and chocolate-chip cookies can enhance anyone's nutrition.

HUMMUS

3 cups canned chickpeas, drained
3 medium cloves garlic
1 ½ tsp. salt
juice of 2 medium lemons
¼ cup chopped parsley (packed)
¼ cup chopped scallions
¼ cup tahini (sesame butter)

Blend all ingredients except tahini in a blender or food processor. Add water as needed to form a thick paste. Put in a bowl and stir in tahini. Chill. Serve on sandwiches or as a dip. Delicious with pita bread and cut vegetables, such as carrots and celery.

PINTO BEAN SPREAD

2 cups canned pinto beans, drained
¾ tsp. garlic powder
½ Tbsp. onion powder
¼–½ tsp. cumin
¼ cup canola oil
½–1 tsp. salt, to taste
dash of black pepper, to taste

Process all ingredients in a blender until smooth. Use on nachos, tacos, and burritos. Top with salsa, avocado, olives, tomatoes, lettuce, and the like.

Courtesy of the North American Vegetarian Society

Seaview Salsa

    5 tomatoes
    1 large onion
  10 sprigs flat leaf parsley
    1 fresh green chile

Chop all ingredients by hand and combine in a bowl. Toss and serve with tortilla chips.

Courtesy of Michael Frank

Guacamole

    3 very ripe avocados
    2 large tomatoes
    1 medium onion
     several sprigs cilantro
     salt and pepper, to taste

Peel avocados, remove pits, and mash in a medium bowl. Chop onion and cilantro and mix well into avocado. Add salt and pepper as desired. Serve with tortilla chips.

Courtesy of Deborah Donenfeld

ENGLISH MUFFIN PIZZAS

English muffins
pizza sauce
mozzarella cheese, grated*
assorted vegetables (optional) †

Preheat oven or toaster oven to 350°F. In a toaster oven, use "top broil" after pizzas are cooked.

Spread pizza sauce on English muffin halves. Sprinkle grated cheese over sauce. Bake until cheese is melted and muffins are toasted.

*If you want to make this a vegan snack, omit the cheese and check store-bought English muffins to ensure that they are not made with eggs or dairy products.
†Any toppings you like on regular pizza are great on these as well; for example, black olives, onions, mushrooms, green peppers, and the like.

VEGETARIAN TACOS

    1 dozen taco shells
    2 tomatoes, chopped
    1 head of iceberg lettuce, shredded
    ½ lb. cheddar cheese, shredded, *or*
      soy cheese
    1 pint plain nonfat yogurt
      guacamole (optional)
    6 cakes ground tofu *or* 16 oz.
      textured vegetable protein (TVP)
    1 Tbsp. vegetable oil
    1 tsp. cumin
    ½ tsp. chili powder
      salt and pepper, to taste

Preheat oven to 250°F.

Place taco shells on a baking sheet and set aside.

Put tomatoes, lettuce, cheese, yogurt, and guacamole in separate bowls.

Fry tofu in oil in a wok or frying pan with oil. Add cumin, chili powder, salt, and pepper just as tofu is becoming crispy. Simmer for 10 minutes. Remove from heat.

Heat taco shells in oven for 5 minutes.

Stuff taco shells with a heaping tablesoon of tofu and whatever other ingredients you like. Top with Taco Sauce, yogurt, and guacamole.

Taco Sauce

3 ripe tomatoes, puréed
1 green bell pepper, chopped
1 green chile, minced
1 small onion, chopped

Mix all ingredients together in a blender. Sauce should have a chunky consistency.

12 servings.

CARROT PATÉ

1 large carrot, peeled and chopped
1 tsp. olive oil
1 ½ cups onion, minced
1 tsp. dried thyme
1 tsp. dried basil
1 ½ cups leftover cooked beans and
grains, such as:
brown rice
millet
lentils
chickpeas
split peas
lima beans
or a combination of any of these
salt and pepper, to taste

Cook the carrots in enough water to cover until very soft.
Drain; save water. Set aside.

Heat olive oil in a skillet. Add onions and dried herbs. Cook
until onions are very soft and golden.

Purée the carrots with ½ cup of the water they were cooked
in and the rest of the ingredients.

Spread on fresh bread as a snack or serve in pita bread with
veggies and sprouts.

Courtesy of Chef Jeanette Maier

BAKED POTATO CHIPS

6 large potatoes
2 Tbsp. olive oil
    salt and paprika, to taste

Preheat oven to 400°F.

Peel potatoes and cut into thin slices. If you have a food processor, use the slicing blade.

Place slices on a baking sheet. Sprinkle with olive oil, salt, and a little paprika.

Bake until crispy. Eat as an alternative to fried potato chips.

POPCORN MEDLEY

½ cup popping corn
½ tsp. salt
½ tsp. pepper
¼ tsp. chili pepper
¼ tsp. garlic powder
½ tsp. vegetable oil

Pop corn in air popper.

Place all seasonings, oil, and popcorn in a plastic bag and toss.

Add other spices according to taste.

TRAIL MIX

You can make trail mix from almost anything, adding and
omitting whatever you choose. Some suggestions
include:

> peanuts
> sesame sticks
> chocolate chips
> banana chips
> dried apricots, apples, pears
> prunes
> walnuts
> Brazil nuts
> hazelnuts
> sunflower seeds
> pumpkin seeds
> Cornnuts

Trail mix is great for energy boosts at school, at home, or out
on the trail. A lot of the nuts and seeds have other nutrients that you need each day, making trail mix a healthy
alternative to candy, but do not gorge on it, as it is usually
very high in calories and fat.

VEGGIE BURGERS

Veggie burgers make great meals as well as snacks. Following are some points that will make them more enjoyable and healthy:

◇ Veggie burgers tend to be very fast to make and quite nutritious.

◇ Try not to fry them, but broil and grill them when you can, to avoid extra fat from cooking oil.

◇ There are many different kinds on the market. Try several to find the ones you like best.

◇ You can eat veggie burgers just like beef and turkey burgers, with lettuce, tomato, ketchup, and mustard. You can also try different condiments and vegetables, such as relish and red peppers.

Listed below are some popular brands of veggie burgers you may want to try:

◇ Boca Burgers

◇ Natural Touch Okra Patty

◇ GardenChef Paul Wenner's Veggie Gardenburger

OTHER SNACKS

Some other good-tasting vegetarian snack products are:

◇Cheese: Soymage Soy Singles, Rice Slice, and SoyaKaas

◇*Hot Dogs*: Yves chili and hot dogs and Lightlife Smart Dogs

◇Yves veggie bacon and Lightlife sausage

◇Lightlife Tempeh: Indonesian soy food that is high in protein and can be used much like tofu and as a good meat alternative. Use in stir-fries and on sandwiches.

TIME TO EAT

ONCE YOU BECOME comfortable in the kitchen, there will be no end to what you can create. It is helpful to think of cooking as a creative act, one that directly benefits you and your family. Melissa Smith says, "Once I began making vegetarian food, my whole family started eating a healthier diet." Preparing vegetarian meals may take a little longer than throwing a hamburger in a frying pan and some french fries in the oven, but you will be amazed at the variety of tastes available to you.

Now that you are on your way to becoming a confident chef, you may want to find out more about vegetarian cooking and what other people are whipping up. You may also be curious about how to get in touch with other teenage vegetarians across the country and find out about events in your area. In the final chapter, you will find information about organizations, groups, magazines, articles, and Internet forums that give you access to a community full of welcoming vegetarian teens.

7

WHERE TO FIND IT:
RESOURCES FOR THE VEGETARIAN TEENAGER

*Ask, and it shall be given you; seek
and ye shall find; knock, and it shall
be opened unto you.*

—Matthew 7:7

VEGETARIANISM is on the rise, especially among teenagers. There are literally millions of vegetarians in the United States and many have questions and concerns about what it means to stop cosuming meat and, in some cases, animal products altogether. In response to this vegetarian explosion, people have created groups, written books, and started magazines, all focusing on the subject and lending support to the converted.

If a national organization seems too impersonal and far away for you, try starting an animal rights group or vegetarian club at your school. You can begin by focusing on the treatment of animals, one of the primary reasons that teens become vegetarians. Other goals can include working toward the establishment of a healthy lunch program and raising awareness about vegetarianism without beating people over the head with it.

Knowing where to find good vegetarian food, either at a health food store or a restaurant, is also very useful when your parents throw up their hands in frustration. With your new recipes and some fresh ingredients, you can prepare dinner for the family one night during the week. Everyone in the family

will get to try something new and your parents will be happy
to see that you are making an effort toward taking responsibility for your own nutrition.

Whatever you decide, use the information in this chapter
when you feel the need to connect with others who know
what it is like being a vegetarian in a meat-based culture.

ORGANIZATIONS

**The American Dietetic Association Consumer
Nutrition Hotline**
800-366-1655 (toll free)
Office hours are 9 A.M. to 4 P.M. Central Time, Monday
through Friday
Dietitians will answer your questions on general nutrition.

The American Vegan Society
501 Old Harding Highway
Malaga, NJ 08328
609-694-2887
This society answers questions and offers support about an
animal product–free lifestyle for both adults and children.
Hosts a biennial conference on veganism and publishes a
newsletter called *Ahimsa*.

Animalearn
801 Old York Road #204
Jenkintown, PA 19046-1685
215-887-0816
An animal rights group that provides information for students. Also offers summer programs and workshops for
kids.

Center for Science in the Public Interest
1875 Connecticut Avenue, NW
Suite 300
Washington, DC 20009-5278
202-332-9110
This group provides ample and truthful nutritional information about food. Sponsors and runs a campaign for kids called "Kids Against Junk Food," and publishes the *Nutrition Action Newsletter*.

Dissection Hotline
run by the North American Vegetarian Society
609-694-2887
Gives advice to students who do not want to participate in animal dissection in school.

EarthSave Foundation International
706 Frederick Street
Santa Cruz, CA 96062-2205
408-423-4069
Sponsors of the Healthy School Lunch Program. An environmental organization that focuses on how changes in dietary habits can change the planet. Founded by John Robbins, author of *Diet for a New America*. A good source of information on how vegetarianism is good for the planet.

Farm Sanctuary
P.O. Box 150
Watkins Glen, NY 14891
607-583-2225
This farm literally provides a sanctuary and home for animals rescued from factory farms. For interested teens, Farm Sanctuary has internships in New York and California.

**Interfaith Council for the Protection of Animals and
  Nature**
4290 Raintree Lane, NW
Atlanta, GA 30327
404-252-9176
Provides information about vegetarianism and world religions. Also discusses how religion can play a role in protecting animals.

The North American Vegetarian Society
P.O. Box 52
Dolgeville, NY 13329
518-568-7970
Established in 1975, this society publishes a magazine called *Vegetarian Voice* and sponsors local chapters. Holds Summerfest, an annual educational and recreational conference for families. Provides ample literature on nutrition, support, and updated information about vegetarianism.

People for the Ethical Treatment of Animals (PETA)
501 Front Street
Norfolk, VA 23510
757-622-7382
Promotes the welfare and proper treatment of animals. Has a vegetarian program for kids and provides ample literature on vegetarian issues.

Physicians' Committee for Responsible Medicine
P.O. Box 96736
Washington, DC 20090-6736
202-686-2210
Promotes a total vegetarian diet and alternatives to lab testing on animals. Publishes a journal called *Good Medicine* and a useful booklet for new vegetarians. Good resource for asking medical questions that your doctor may be unable to answer.

Students for the Ethical Treatment of Animals (SETA)
715 Stadium Drive
P.O. Box 1187
Trinity University
San Antonio, TX 78212-7200
512-737-4237
Student group that promotes the ethical treatment of animals, often adopting cows and chickens, and encourages a vegetarian lifestyle for teens.

The Vegetarian Education Network
P.O. Box 339
Oxford, PA 19363-0339
717-529-8638
An organization founded by Sally Clinton expressly to meet the needs of young vegetarians. Sponsors school forums and travel to foreign countries, publishes the magazine *How on Earth!* (written by young people ages 13 to 24), and provides lots of literature as well as advice on the phone. Excellent resource.

The Vegetarian Resource Group
P.O. Box 1463
Baltimore, MD 21203
410-366-8343

Provides great educational programs and information on the latest scientific findings about vegetarianism. Publishes several books and the magazine *Vegetarian Journal*. Their 112-page book, *Vegetarian Journal Reports*, features, among other things, a 28-day meal plan, recipes, a weight-loss guide, information for athletes, healthy food substitutes, a hospital survival guide, and a list of where to find nonleather shoes.

FURTHER READING

As I MENTIONED before, books are a great place to discover why vegetarianism makes so much sense for you personally as well as for the health of the planet. With so many teens and others joining the ranks of vegetarians, there is a seemingly never-ending supply of both informational books and cookbooks available. The following are a few selections worth investigating.

GENERAL READING

Becoming Vegetarian: The Complete Guide to Adopting a Healthy Vegetarian Diet, by Vesanto Melina, RD, Brenda Davis, RD., and Victoria Harrison, RD. Summertown, TN: Book Publishing Company, 1995.

Beyond Beef, by Jeremy Rifkin. New York: Dutton, 1992.

Conscious Eating, by Gabriel Cousens, M.D. Patagonia, AZ: Essene Vision Books, 1995.

Diet for a New America: How Your Food Choices Affect Your Health, Happiness and the Future of Life on Earth, by John Robbins. Walpole, NH: Stillpoint Publishing, 1987.

Diet for a Small Planet, 20th Anniversary Edition, by Frances Moore Lappé. New York: Ballantine Books, 1991.

Dr. Attwood's Low-Fat Prescription for Kids: A Pediatrician's Program of Preventive Nutrition, by Charles R. Attwood, M.D. New York: Viking, 1995.

For the Vegetarian in You, by Billy Ray Boyd. Santa Cruz, CA: Taterhill, 1987.

The Healthy School Action Guide, by Susan Campbell and Todd Winant. Santa Cruz, CA: EarthSave Foundation, 1994.

The Jungle, by Upton Sinclair. Ask at your bookstore or library for the most recent edition.

May All Be Fed, by John Robbins. New York: William Morrow, 1992.

Vegan Nutrition: Pure and Simple, by Michael Klaper, M.D. Umatilla, FL: Gentle World, 1987.

The Vegetarian Alternative: A Guide to a Healthful and Humane Diet, by Vic Sussman. Emmaus, PA: Rodale Press, 1978.

The Vegetarian Handbook: Eating Right for Total Health, by Gary Null. New York: St. Martin's Press, 1987.

The Vegetarian Way: Total Health for You and Your Family, by Virginia Messina, MPH, RD and Mark Messina, Ph.D. New York: Crown Trade Paperbacks, 1996.

Vegetarianism: A Way of Life, by Dudley Giehl. New York: Harper & Row, 1979.

COOKBOOKS

All the Best Potatoes, by Joie Warner. New York: Hearst Books, 1993.

All the Best Stir-Fries, by Joie Warner. New York: Hearst Books, 1993.

The Burrito Book, by P. J. Birosik. New York: Avon Books, 1991.

The Compassionate Cook, by People for the Ethical Treatment of Animals and Ingrid Newkirk. New York: Warner Books, 1993.

The Enchanted Broccoli Forest, by Mollie Katzen. Berkeley, CA: Ten Speed Press, 1995.

The Moosewood Cookbook, by Mollie Katzen. Berkeley, CA: Ten Speed Press, 1992.

The Natural Gourmet, by Annemarie Colbin. New York: Ballantine Books, 1989.

The New Basics Cookbook, by Julee Rosso and Sheila Lukins. New York: Workman Publishing, 1989.

The New Farm Vegetarian Cookbook, edited by Louise Hagler and Dorothy R. Bates. Summertown, TN: Book Publishing Company, 1988.

New Recipes for Young Vegetarians, by Sammy Green. London: Foulsham, 1988.

New Vegetarian Cuisine, by Linda Rosenweig and the food editors of *Prevention* magazine. Emmaus, PA: Rodale Press, 1994.

Simply Vegan: Quick Vegetarian Meals, by Debra Wasserman and Reed Mangels, Ph.D., RD. Baltimore, MD: Vegetarian Resource Group, 1991.

Still Life with Menu, by Mollie Katzen. Berkeley, CA: Ten Speed Press, 1988.

The Vegetarian Lunchbasket, by Linda Haynes. Willow Springs, MO: Nucleus Publishing, 1990.

Vegetariana: A Rich Harvest of Wit, Lore and Recipes, by Nava Atlas. Garden City, NY: The Dial Press, 1984.

MAGAZINES

Ahimsa, published quarterly by the American Vegan Society, 5501 Harding Highway, Malaga, NJ 08328.

The Environmental Magazine, published bimonthly by the Earth Action Network, 28 Knight Street, Norwalk, CT 06851. Subscription orders: 800-825-0061.

EarthSave, published quarterly by EarthSave Foundation, 706 Frederick Street, Santa Cruz, CA 95062-2205.

How on Earth!, published quarterly by the Vegetarian Education Network, P.O. Box 339, Oxford, PA 19363-0339.

Natural Health, 17 Station Street, Brookline Village, MA 02147. Natural foods, alternative medicine, and nutrition information.

Vegetarian Gourmet, P.O. Box 7641, Riverton, NJ 08077-7641.

Vegetarian Journal, published bimonthly by the Vegetarian Resource Group, P.O. Box 1463, Baltimore, MD 21203.

Vegetarian Times, P.O. Box 570, Oak Park, IL 60303. Subscription orders: 800-435-9610.

Vegetarian Voice, published quarterly by the North American Vegetarian Society, P.O. Box 72, Dolgeville, NY 13329.

Veggie Life, 1401 Shary Circle, Concord, CA 95418.

Articles

Bittman, Mark. "I Was a Teen-Age Vegetarian," *New York Times Magazine*, October 3, 1993, p. 63.

Black, Rosemary. "Vegetarian Generation," *Daily News*, September 21, 1994, Food section, p. 1.

Boccella, Kathy. "When Youngsters Are Fed Up with Meat, Woe to Families," *Philadelphia Inquirer*, October 22, 1995, p. A1.

Gaines, Judith. "Vegetarians Sprouting Up," *Boston Globe*, October 23, 1994, p. 1

Kaufman, Leslie. "Children of the Corn," *Newsweek*, August 28, 1995, pp. 60–62.

Moran, Victoria. "Getting Started as a Vegetarian Family," *Mothering*, September 30, 1996, pp. 64–72.

Nhu, T. T. "The Children Who Won't Eat Their Meat," *San Jose Mercury News*, July 24, 1994, p. 2H.

Pappano, Laura. "Teens Who Go Green," *Boston Globe*, September 30, 1992, Food section.

Reinan, John. "Animal Attraction," (Rochester, NY) *Democrat and Chronicle*, August 28, 1995, p. 6C.

Salomon, Debbie. "Meet the New Vegetarians," *Burlington (VT) Free Press*, February 22, 1994, p. 1D.

Stearns, Patty LaNoue. "Vegging Out," *Detroit Free Press*, May 5, 1995, p. 1F.

Vivinetto, Gina. "I Was a Teenage Vegan," *St. Petersburg Times*, February 13, 1994, p. 13F.

VIDEOS

All the videotapes listed below are available from *Vegetarian Voice*, c/o North American Vegetarian Society, Box 72, Dolgeville, NY 13329; 518-568-7970.

Diet for a New America: Your Health, Your Planet.

This hour-long tape is based on John Robbins's revealing and informative book.

Friendly Foods Gourmet Vegetarian Cuisine: A Cooking Training Video.

By Brother Ron Pickarski. Helps get you started as a vegetarian chef, including step-by-step procedures.

Good Food Today, Great Kids Tomorrow: Jay Gordon, M.D., Talks to Parents about Kids and Food.

Even though this tape is geared toward parents, it is good for you to also hear the issues that concern them.

The Healthy Vegetarian: A Guide to Becoming a Vegetarian.

This 70-minute video explains the *whys* and *hows* of vegetarianism.

Jay Gordon Talks to Kids about Food.

A lively video with discussions about junk food, health, school lunch, self-esteem, peer pressure, and other hot topics for teens.

DINING AND TRAVEL GUIDES

ALL OF THESE guides are available through *Vegetarian Voice*, c/o North American Vegetarian Society, Box 72, Dolgeville, NY 13329; 518-568-7970.

> If you visit Canada, *The Canadian Vegetarian Dining Guide: Your Passport to Healthy Eating in Canada*, by Lynne Tomlinson, is an excellent resource. The guide lists more than 250 places to eat in Canada.

> Plan on traveling to Asia? *Vegetarian Asia: A Travel Guide*, by Teresa Bergen, gives you dining tips, advice on food customs, language hints, and much more to make your trip easier.

> An ultimate source for travel in both the United States and Canada is *The Vegetarian Journal's Guide to Natural Food Restaurants in the United States and Canada*. It includes over 1,300 places to dine and offers both ideas for travel and camping.

COLLEGES

MANY TEENAGE VEGETARIANS are concerned that when they go to college, finding palatable meatless meals will become an impossible task. Most college food services have salad bars, but how much salad can you eat? One thing to do is call ahead, before freshman orientation, and find out the possibilities. Some schools have already made great leaps toward offering serious vegetarian fare. Listed here are a few of the best.

College of the Atlantic (COA)
Bar Harbor, ME 04609
207-288-5015

COA is an alternative school of about 250 students that offers only one undergraduate degree in what they call "Human Ecology." It offers vegetarian entrées at every meal, and vegan meals are often part of the fare. The meal plan was once all vegetarian, but the college does not want to discriminate against anyone, so it now includes meat dishes on the menu.

The College of Wooster
Wooster, OH 44691
800-877-9905

At this school of 1,700 students, vegetarian entrées are served at every meal. Wooster food service also usually includes some vegan side dishes. However, there are not enough vegan options to constitute an entire meal. The college has several different environmental groups and a required Independent Study program in which all juniors and seniors participate.

Oberlin College
Office of Admissions
Carnegie Building
101 N. Professor Street
Oberlin, OH 44074-1075

Oberlin offers a program called the Co-ops, which provide students with an alternative meal/housing plan. One Co-op is entirely vegetarian and another is all vegan. The Co-ops save students about $450 a month and ask for only four to six hours of work a week. The work may entail washing dishes, light cleaning, and other household tasks. Oberlin is home to several active campus organizations, including Oberlin Animal Rights and Oberlin College Habitat for Humanity (a group that builds houses for people without homes).

INTERNET GROUPS

THE REGIONAL VEG NETWORK

The Internet has branched out to touch almost every aspect of our lives in just a short amount of time. This includes vegetarianism. If you have a computer and Internet access, then you can log on to the RegionalVeg Network and join an ongoing discussion of regional vegetarian topics and concerns. RegionalVeg hopes to create forums to explore local issues, which are not provided by larger vegetarian resources on the Internet.

If you want to know more about what is happening with vegetarianism in your area, then RegionalVeg is your site. The enormous mailing list aims to share information about restaurants, stores, events, and any other activities in your area. Because the focus of this group is so specific, it is ideal for online teens who want to know more about vegetarianism in their immediate area.

Some of the areas that are currently part of the RegionalVeg Network are:

◆ Veg-Boston
◆ Veg-CT

◇Veg-FL

◇Veg-LA

◇Veg-NY

◇Veg-OH

◇Veg-WV

and many other states. If you are interested in joining, send an e-mail message to **waste@waste.org** with one of the following commands in the message:

◇subscribe veg-[region] (for normal version)

◇subscribe veg-[region]-digest (for the digest version)

If you find there is no list for your region, you can help the Network create one.

You can also help the RegionalVeg project by creating and owning new lists, administering list software, and coordinating with other vegetarian resources.

Veg-Teen

This group lends support through a chat line for vegetarian teens. They encourage discussion of all topics relating to teenage vegetarianism and vegetarianism in general.

To subscribe, send an e-mail message to: **listproc @envirolink.org** with the following command in the message:

◇subscribe veg-teen [Your Name]

GETTING THE MOST FROM THE VEGETARIAN MARKET

THERE ARE MANY places to find food and other products for your new vegetarian lifestyle. Listed here are both specific and general resources and information that you will need to investigate further to see if they meet your needs. Vegetarian organizations and Internet groups, such as the RegionalVeg Network, are excellent tools to use in your search for the freshest, healthiest, and most ecologically sustainable foods.

FARMERS' MARKETS

Most major American cities now have farmers' market programs. Small and local farmers truck their produce and goods in from the country and sell them out of small stalls. The food tends to be organic and usually very fresh. The money you spend goes directly to the farm and not to some enormous conglomerate. If you are not aware of a farmers' market in your area, call your chamber of commerce or city hall and ask about starting up a program. Markets tend to be visually appealing, with bins of fresh and colorful vegetables, fruits, and flowers. Many also sell baked goods, honeys, jams, organic meats, and dairy products.

NATURAL FOOD STORES

Even if you are not aware of it, you are probably not too far from a natural food store. The phone book is a good place to look, or ask some of your vegetarian (or nonvegetarian) friends if they know of one nearby. Health food stores tend to carry the veggie burgers and hot dogs you may want to try, as well as natural cereals and grains, produce, cosmetics not tested on animals, and delicious fruit juices. Unfortunately, because they are not national chains, the products tend to be a little more expensive than those in supermarkets. However, as more people demand ecologically sustainable and organic goods, more national chains are opening—for example, General Nutrition Centers (GNC). As a greater number of people demand vegetarian and organic choices, the price of such items as Boca Burgers and SoyaKaas cheese will begin to fall as more places carry them.

FOOD CO-OPS

Food co-ops have been around for a long time and continue to be a great place to find everything you need for your vegetarian diet. Most require a little bit of your time each month, but it is a small price to pay for the high quality and the low prices. Co-ops can keep prices very low because they buy in bulk and then sell the goods at nearly wholesale prices. They also do not have to pay employees because the work is all done by co-op members. Again, to find out if there is a food co-op near you, look in the phone book, ask around, or log on to the Internet for information.

BUY IN BULK

A great way to ensure that you will have enough vegetarian food and keep the bills low is to buy in bulk. Most grains, nuts, seeds, and certain vegetables, such as potatoes and squashes, will stay fresh for long periods of time if kept in cool, dry settings. Buying in bulk also ensures that you will always have something on hand to cook for dinner or snack on in the middle of the afternoon.

GO ETHNIC

A great way to perk up dishes you create in the kitchen is to use ethnic ingredients. If your area has a Middle Eastern or Asian food market, try some of the spices, grains, and produce available at these stores to add new dimensions to your cooking. Also investigate ethnic restaurants near you. Do not overlook Ethiopian, Vietnamese, Thai, Japanese, Mexican, Chinese, and Middle Eastern establishments, which offer many different vegetarian dishes.

VEGETARIAN COOKING CLASS

If you have the time and the interest, try taking a vegetarian cooking class at a nearby school or institute. Cooking classes are a lot of fun, and you will be amazed how much you can learn in a weekend. You will gain new confidence in the kitchen as well as a new appreciation for the huge variety inherent in vegetarian cuisine. Your parents will probably also be impressed by your commitment to learning about vegetarian fare. Offer to prepare a meal for them once the class is over. Better yet, see if one of them wants to take the class with you.

ANIMAL-FREE SHOPPING

A lot of teenage vegetarians want to stop buying clothes and other products that are made from or tested on animals or that are harmful to the environment. Many companies that are ecologically and animal friendly advertise in the back of vegetarian and environmental magazines. *Vegetarian Times* has a wonderful section in the main body of the magazine called "Shopping Around," which features new and innovative vegetarian products and where to find and order them.

Organizations usually have extensive lists of places to order anything from bleach-free cotton to dairyless cheese to non-leather shoes and bags.

The National Organic Directory, a 404-page tome that contains more than 2,000 listings of wholesalers and organic farmers who sell directly to the public, is an excellent place to begin your shopping. It is available from Community Alliance with Family Farmers, P.O. Box 464, Davis, CA 95617. You can also order by phone at 800-852-3832. The directory costs $34.95 (plus $5.50 shipping and handling).

TRY EVERYTHING

I STRONGLY ENCOURAGE you to use all the resources available to you. When you first become a vegetarian, you'll probably still have some lingering questions. Don't panic if at first you can't find a particular answer. As you have heard from the many voices in this book, there is a community out there ready to address your concerns and embrace you with open arms. Ideally, you will be improving your health, as well as helping animals and the environment. In addition, with a little perseverance and patience, you will also start to discover a world of other vegetarians eager to share their experiences and help make the transition for you not only simple, but enjoyable.

Glossary

amino acids: The building blocks of protein. There are 22 amino acids, 8 of which are essential to human beings.

anemia: An oxygen deficiency in the blood, generally due to low iron, which makes people weak and listless.

enzymes: Catalysts for chemical reactions in living organisms. The enzyme lactase aids with the digestion of lactose, the sugar in milk.

ethics: A principle of good or correct behavior. If you have a good sense of ethics, you generally make decisions based on morally upstanding ideas.

high blood pressure: A condition in which the pressure of the blood within your arteries and veins becomes elevated because your blood vessels have become partially blocked. The result is that the same amount of blood is now trying to move through a much smaller space. As a result, pressure increases throughout the system, placing strain on your blood vessels and heart. Partially clogged plumbing pipes are a good metaphor for high blood pressure.

hormone: A substance produced in the body by one organ

that acts on another organ or system of organs elsewhere in the body.

livestock: Animals, such as cows, pigs, sheep, or chickens, raised for home use or slaughter. Animals bred and owned by the meat and dairy industries are livestock.

Methodism: A denomination of Protestant Christianity. John and Charles Wesley, and others in England, developed Methodist ideas in the early part of the eighteenth century. The religion is based on doctrines of free grace and individual responsibility.

pesticides: Chemical agents used by farmers to kill insects and rodents harmful to their crops. Residues from the pesticides can remain on the crops and are passed along to those who eat them.

Seventh-Day Adventists: Members of a branch of Christianity begun by Ellen White in the 1840s. The church differs from most other denominations in that its members observe the Sabbath on Saturday rather than Sunday. Many Seventh-Day Adventists are vegetarians, as they focus on spiritual health achieved in part by diet and exercise.

tubers: Potatoes, turnips, sweet potatoes, and radishes are all examples of tubers, vegetables that grow from an underground stem and from which new plant shoots arise.

vegan: A type of vegetarian who consumes no animal food or dairy products. Many vegans also refuse to use any products that come from animals, such as feathers, leather, and wool.

Notes

Introduction:
1. Charles R. Attwood. *Dr. Attwood's Low-Fat Prescription for Kids: A Pediatrician's Program of Preventive Nutrition* (New York: Viking, 1995), p.4.

2. Marianne Rackliffe. "Diet Clash," *How on Earth!* Spring/Early Summer 1995, Issue #10, p.13.

Chapter 1:
1. Virginia Messina, MPH, RD, and Mark Messina, Ph.D., *The Vegetarian Way: Total Health for You and Your Family* (New York: Crown Trade Paperbacks, 1996), p. 9.

2. Gary Null. *The Vegetarian Handbook: Eating Right for Total Health* (New York: St. Martin's Press, 1987), p. 12.

3. Dudley Giehl. *Vegetarianism: A Way of Life* (New York: Harper & Row, 1979), p. 134.

4. Ibid., p. 139.

Chapter 2:

1. Leslie Kaufman. "Children of the Corn," *Newsweek*, August 28, 1995, p. 60.

2. Rosemary Black. "Vegetarian Generation," *Daily News*, (New York) September 21, 1994, Food section, p. 1.

3. John Robbins. *Diet for a New America: How Your Food Choices Affect Your Health, Happiness and the Future of Life on Earth* (Walpole, NH: Stillpoint Publishing, 1987), p. 111.

4. L. Taylor. *National Hog Farmer*, March 1978, p. 27.

5. Sue Coe. *Dead Meat* (New York: Four Walls Eight Windows, 1996), p. 69.

6. Kaufman, p. 60.

7. Vesanto Melina, RD, Brenda Davis, RD, and Victoria Harrison, RD, *Becoming Vegetarian: The Complete Guide to Adopting a Healthy Vegetarian Diet* (Summertown, TN: Book Publishing Company, 1995), p. 21.

8. Null, p. 34.

9. Ibid., p. 165.

10. Robbins, pp. 350–351.

11. Ibid., p. 353.

12. Frances Moore Lappé. *Diet for a Small Planet* (New York: Ballantine, 1982), p. 66.

13. Giehl, p. 170.

14. Kaufman, p. 60.

15. Sara Gilbert. "A Special Message from Sara," *Tiger Beat*, October, 1993.

16. Gina Vivinetto. "I Was a Teenage Vegan," *St. Petersburg Times*, February 13, 1994, p. 3F.

17. Annie Nakao. "Veggie Kids: The Young and the Fleshless," *San Francisco Examiner*, April 12, 1994, p. B4.

18. Judith Gaines. "Vegetarians Sprouting Up," *Boston Globe*, October 23, 1994, p.1.

19. Virginia Baldwin Hick. "Vegetarians of Tender Years on the Rise," *St. Louis Post-Dispatch*, October 3, 1993, p. 5.

20. Gaines, p. 1.

21. Nakao, p. B-4.

22. Null, p. 101.

23. Vic Sussman. *The Vegetarian Alternative: A Guide to a Healthful and Humane Diet* (Emmaus, PA: Rodale Press, 1978), p. 48.

24. Ibid.

25. Kaufman, p. 61.

26. Ibid., p. 62.

Chapter 3
1. Giehl, p. 4.

2. Messina, p. 18.

3. Vivinetto, p. 3F.

4. Debbie Salomon. "Meet the New Vegetarians," *Burlington Free Press*, (Burlington, VT) February, 22, 1994.

5. Ibid.

Chapter 4:
1. Robbins, p. 159.

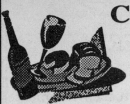

Cookbooks for Vegetarians

from the

Berkley Publishing Group

___VEGETARIAN COOKING by Louise Pickford
                          1-557-88076-X/$12.00

___THE PRACTICALLY MEATLESS GOURMET
      by Cornelia Carlson   0-425-15131-X/$12.00

___THE VEGETARIAN CHILD by Lucy Moll
                          0-399-52271-9/$12.00

___THE NO-TOFU VEGETARIAN COOKBOOK
      by Sharon Sassaman Claessens
                          1-55788-269-X/$14.00

VISIT THE PUTNAM BERKLEY BOOKSTORE CAFÉ ON THE INTERNET:
http://www.berkley.com

Payable in U.S. funds. No cash accepted. Postage & handling: $1.75 for one book, 75¢ for each additional. Maximum postage $5.50. Prices, postage and handling charges may change without notice. Visa, Amex, MasterCard call 1-800-788-6262, ext. 1, or fax 1-201-933-2316; refer to ad #745

Or, check above books   Bill my: ☐ Visa ☐ MasterCard ☐ Amex _____ (expires)
and send this order form to:
The Berkley Publishing Group   Card#_____
                                                                   ($10 minimum)
P.O. Box 12289, Dept. B   Daytime Phone #_____
Newark, NJ 07101-5289   Signature_____
Please allow 4-6 weeks for delivery.   Or enclosed is my: ☐ check ☐ money order
Foreign and Canadian delivery 8-12 weeks.
Ship to:
Name_____   Book Total $_____
Address_____   Applicable Sales Tax $_____
                                         (NY, NJ, PA, CA, GST Can.)
City_____   Postage & Handling $_____
State/ZIP_____   Total Amount Due $_____
Bill to: Name_____
Address_____City_____
State/ZIP_____